FITNESS HOLLYWOOD

KELI ROBERTS

**The Trainer
to the
STARS
Shares Her
Body-Shaping
Secrets**

Fitness

Hollywood

THE SUMMIT GROUP ❧ FORT WORTH, TEXAS

THE SUMMIT GROUP

1227 West Magnolia, Suite 500 • Fort Worth, Texas 76102

Printed in the United States of America.

95 96 97 98 99   5 4 3 2 1

The suggestions for stretching, exercise, weight training, and all other health-and-fitness-related subjects in this book are not intended as a substitute for consultation with a fitness instructor and/or physician. Before starting any aspect of the Keli Roberts Fitness Hollywood program, you are advised to consult your physician or a qualified health professional for specific guidance. The mention of specific products in this book does not constitute an endorsement by the publisher.

Library of Congress Cataloging-in-Publication Data

Roberts, Keli, 1961-
    Fitness Hollywood: the trainer to the stars shares her body shaping secrets / Keli Roberts.
        p.cm.
    Includes bibliographical references and index.
    ISBN 1-56530-147-1: $19.95
    1. Exercise. 2. Health. 3. Physical fitness. I. Title.
RA781.R62 1994   94-23938
613.7—dc20   CIP

Cover design by David Sims
Book design by Sean Walker
Cover and inside photography by Roni Ramos

To all my clients and students,
who inspire and motivate me and from whom I learn so much.

Contents

9   STRENGTH-TRAINING EXERCISES: *UPPER BODY*...................225

Preface

Loving yourself begins with being courteous… if we've been hating ourselves, we need to begin slowly changing that idea, through changing our actions. Actions speak louder than words; by taking loving or courteous actions toward our body, mind, and soul, we can begin that process in a very tangible and practical manner.
—Keli Roberts

I kept getting the message early in my life from a number of sources that it was wrong to be me, that there was something very wrong about being as tall and as muscular as I was as a teenager, and that in order to be acceptable, I had to be at least twenty-two pounds lighter, and delicate and fragile looking—feminine in the *Gone with the Wind* style, with the eighteen-inch waist and the willowy female look. But I was an athlete. I was on every school team possible. I was a champion swimmer, high jumper, and gymnast … a bundle of muscle, really fit and very healthy. However, I thought as girls grew into women, they were supposed to inherit their mother's body. Somehow, I wound up with a body more like my father's; he was a footballer! While "his body" suited him perfectly, it didn't fit my idea of femininity.

Somewhere in all this, my self-esteem went wacko. When I was fifteen, I began using a lot of drugs and alcohol. As soon as I left school, my substance abuse severely escalated to the point of heavy daily use. My awareness of weight control and thinness began at about age sixteen because all the girls my age seemed to be completely absorbed in dieting. It was the "thing to do," to worry about weight, and discuss dieting plans and pounds lost or gained. I wanted so much to fit in that I went on a diet, even though I had absolutely no excess weight to lose. I didn't even really associate dieting with weight loss, it was just something that everybody was doing, and I wanted to be a part of it. It was then magnified many times over when my mother got me involved in modeling. The photographers said I had potential, but that I needed to lose at least ten pounds. I was already eating in a disordered, binge-diet mode; but as a result of the added pressure, I became bulimic.

I remember feeling how smart I was because I could just eat huge amounts of food and then throw it back up, not gaining an ounce and maintaining perfect control over my weight. Very quickly I lost almost thirty pounds. People loved the way I looked: I weighed 110 pounds at a height of five-foot-ten, and personified The Look. The Look was thin and beyond. The more I modeled, the more entangled I became with heavy drugs, including acid, cocaine, heroin, hash, grass—all of which was part of Sydney, Australia's modeling scene.

In an effort to give up vomiting, I ended up severely anorexic; I weighed ninety-five pounds. My life was a total nightmare. I was obsessed with rituals, which consisted of taking cold showers to scrub away "toxins" with hard-bristle brushes, and food obsession—what, when, and how to eat, how to cook it, whom to eat it with, and even how many times to chew it. The rest of my time was spent exercising; first calculating how much more had to done that day to account for anything I had eaten. Every day I would swim a mile, ride my bike for two hours, then do four hours of hard, physical yoga. I was completely and utterly abusive to myself. There was certainly no time left for people, relationships or love, let alone an interest or a hobby which didn't involve food, drugs, or exercise.

After a two-year stint modeling in Europe, my illness progressively worsened because I became bulimic for a time instead of just starving myself. My weight actually increased to 120 pounds, but my agent complained that I was getting too heavy. I was described by magazines as the perfect, healthy role model, which only I knew was a deception. My life was going down the toilet, literally. I was vomiting five to fifteen times a day, both my esophagus and stomach were bleeding, my teeth had worn down to brown stubs from the acid in the vomit, my eyes were puffy and bloodshot, and my face was so swollen, I looked like a chipmunk. I was regularly using heroin and cocaine, and drinking two to three bottles of wine a day, not to mention daily Tequila and beer, and smoking two packs of cigarettes.

I was desperate; I wanted to die and knew I would if something didn't change. The sordid modeling scene in Europe had robbed what little self-esteem I'd had and I knew I had to get back to Australia. It was at that time I read a book about a girl who had recovered from anorexia and bulimia. I knew I needed help and I desperately wanted it. Within a few months, I was sober, drug free, and abstinent from the bulimic habit. I hadn't eaten and digested normally in about eight years and my feelings were raw; I was no longer anesthetized.

My system was such a mess that initially I gained a large amount of weight. I hated the weight gain—it terrified me. I thought no one could possibly like me looking like that. After a couple of relapses, I realized that in order to get well I really had to let go of my body image and get to like myself regardless of weight.

I made the decision that it didn't matter how much I weighed or what people thought about me and how I looked, I just had to learn how to eat, I had to recover, I had to get well. After almost a year, I started getting my life back and much to my surprise, people liked and accepted me just as I was. I didn't have to be perfect. Then one day, I had a rude awakening. I caught my unguarded reflection in a shop window. I saw a fat girl in the same dress. Ouch, that girl was me! I managed to ward off the panicky feelings, rationalizing it was a "fat reflection," until about a week later. I was sitting in a pair of very tight jeans (they used to be my baggies, but I figured they'd shrunk), and I went to tuck in the blousing on my T-shirt when total disgust hit me. It wasn't blousing, it was a roll of fat hanging over the tops of my jeans.

I felt sick; the truth was I'd gained a ton of weight. I'd gone up three or four dress sizes, and none of my clothes fit. I never weighed myself or really took a good look at myself in the mirror. I was in total denial about how I felt about myself. I realized once again that it didn't matter what other people thought of me, it was what I thought of myself. I hated the way I looked and worse still, I hated the way I felt about the way I looked.

Dieting was out of the question and my fear of relapsing was enormous. I knew I had no boundaries when it came to food and body image. I needed to find a gentle way of exercising which didn't involve shiny pink spandex thong leotards, keeping up with everyone else, anything intimidating, or any pressure of any sort. So I went to the pool; a place I felt good. A safe place where I could be facedown in the water, watching the sun being reflected in the pool, my hair fanned out by the water, and blowing bubbles quietly. No one stared at me, and I didn't have to look at anyone.

I could just stroll to the pool and do my twenty laps, freestyle one way, breaststroke the other, and then get out. Initially, it took quite awhile to do the twenty laps, but as my strength improved, I started doing them quite quickly. I started feeling a whole lot better about myself. I really enjoyed the swimming; it stilled my racing mind.

But I had a tough time sticking with it. There were days I would wake up not wanting to go. My head would start: "I'm too tired today," or "I don't have time this morning," or "I'm hungry now, I want to eat something." But if I blew it off in the morning, by four o'clock in the afternoon, I would start asking myself: "Why not?" "Why should I?" "I don't feel like it, so I'm not going to do it anyway." Eventually, I would walk down to the pool, just telling myself to get wet and that would make me feel better.

Once in the water, the bargaining thing would begin: "Just do two laps." Well, that sounded manageable. Then I'd do the two and then two more, then say, "Well, I'll do ten." Then, "Well, I'm here; I might as well do my twenty laps."

It was an insight into just how resistant to feeling good I was. There I was doing an activity that brought so much into my life (it was outdoors ... the sun and water ... the cooling down during summer. I was enjoying it, it made me feel better, and I was looking a whole lot better). Still, it was difficult to stick to any type of routine.

But I kept feeling better and began eating better. My body responded to it, started looking really fit and sharp. I started getting compliments, and I began to enjoy wearing my clothes and going out again. I began to feel confident for the first time in years. True confidence! When I had been overweight, I felt like the invisible little sister in the corner that no one wanted to speak to, and after being used to getting a lot of attention, that caused great shame. As a bulimic, I felt like a fraud.

Ultimately, it's how you feel about yourself that is the important thing. Exercise does, indeed, change the way you look, but it also helps you think about yourself and your body in a really positive way because you're the one taking the action—it's not something that's being done to or for you.

I went back to modeling for about nine months, and for the first time in my life, my skin was glowing, my body was strong looking, and I was at a healthy weight. I was still small, a size four to six, but I was eating and by that time had graduated to doing triathlons. I had bought a bike, and I was running and swimming and occasionally lifting weights, and I was finally strong and healthy. I felt in control.

At a fitting for a prestigious modeling job, there was another girl there. She was skeletal; I saw my old self in her. All the people fitting her were saying how fabulous she was and how incredible she looked and, "Wow! Wasn't she wonderful?" It was disgusting. When I phoned the agency to check my call times, they informed me I'd been canceled from the job because they had said I was too big for the clothes, which wasn't true. Everything fitted loosely, just right. I was so furious, I quit modeling, then and there on the spot. I thought, if that girl is the role model for women and how they should feel about themselves, then I don't want to be part of an industry which promotes such an unhealthy body image. It's hard enough for us to feel good about ourselves, let alone cope with something as unrealistic as that.

I was terribly depressed, I had no idea what I was going to do, but I knew it wouldn't involve fashion or modeling. To cheer me up, a friend took me to her favorite aerobics class with a teacher named Rick. I walked in skeptical and came out converted; the music, the energy, the fun. It was nothing like my previous experiences, struggling physically while trying to follow behind a pink lycra-clad, hysterically smiling maniac! I liked Rick's personality. This time I could keep up; I was fit. By giving up smoking and working out at the correct level for me, it actually became fun. I was hooked. I went back the next day and the next and the next. I couldn't wait for Rick's next class. At a friend's suggestion, I signed up to take the Australian Council for Health, Education, and Recreation course to become an aerobics instructor.

What an experience! I had never thought of myself as intelligent or capable of learning any new skill. At the ripe "old age" of twenty-four, I had felt at a dead end; no qualifications, no education beyond high school. Instead, I found studying the human body mentally stimulating and teaching to be physically challenging. Combining those two elements with something that offered people help was perfect. My self-esteem really started improving when I saw what a difference I could make in people's lives. I'd found my niche; my true passion.

One of my first clients came to me weighing 190 pounds, and unable to walk on a treadmill at three miles an hour without seeing stars and getting dizzy. After a number of months, her fitness level had improved and she'd dropped about thirty-five to forty pounds. She had her whole wardrobe altered, and she started waterskiing, snow skiing, hiking, going on canoeing adventures with people. No longer was she scared to go to barbecues and social events, because she was no longer ashamed of her body.

Her transformation brought back the memory of when life changed for me, remembering when I started feeling good about myself, then realizing I wasn't even aware of just how ashamed I had been until change began to happen. With this newfound consciousness, all of a sudden I was living again, willing to go out dancing and out to dinner because I could make healthy choices in food and clothes, and not feel ashamed of who I was. Body shape had little to do with it; self-worth as a human being did. To be part of stimulating that process for other people is what keeps me interested, motivated, and committed in the fitness industry.

I love watching the changes in people's lives, not just their bodies, as a result of discovering their own internal and external strengths. At one time, I hadn't known it was possible to walk up a flight of stairs without getting out of breath, or carry bags of groceries without feeling like passing out, and it's difficult to describe to someone the joy of becoming strong unless you've had the experience yourself. I love my new lifestyle; as a result of changing my habits, it has truly given me a life.

This doesn't mean you have to be ball-and-chained to dumbbells, incarcerated in a gym to receive the benefits of being fit and healthy. I started out with very little and very quickly got decent results, and so can everyone else. People who keep waiting to start don't have any idea just how good they're going to feel. It's like going to the beach. If you stopped to think about the traffic jam, the heat, and the struggle for the parking space, you would never go. But when people think about how much fun it's going to be—about the swimming and the sipping something cool sitting on the sand, about the refreshing feeling on their skin when they wash the salt off and the fact that when they get home, they're going to feel warm, glowing, relaxed, and healthy—they can't wait to have the next opportunity to go to the beach. When people keep putting off getting started in a fitness routine because they don't have the energy, they don't realize that the exercise will give them the energy—which may be the least understood aspect of exercise by someone who doesn't exercise.

You can start out with little baby steps and discover it gets much easier as you go along. That's the process: just being involved will keep you going because fitness produces so many tangible results—it becomes enjoyable and valuable in and of itself because it makes you feel so good.

Fitness makes my life more productive. You get to take responsibility for yourself by making healthy lifestyle choices. It all begins here, with you. I can't remember the last time I was sick or needed to take antibiotics. The situations we place ourselves in, how we spend our time and energy, ultimately affect not only our bodies, but also our minds and spirits as well. The journey has begun, welcome aboard. Oh, and by the way, if you've taken the scenic route … don't forget to watch for the changing scenery.

I was never born to be a willowy, delicate, little rose. I'm five-foot-ten and 147 pounds of bone and muscle and strength, and that's how I was supposed to be all my life. And the thing I love about my recovery, about learning to eat, to accept myself and work out, is that I am now the person I was always meant to be.

I'm now the ideal representation of me! I feel a real freedom and a great deal of strength from that, and I think that anyone can achieve that, given the willingness to begin. It's not that it's easy. But it's simple—as simple as taking the first step.

—*Keli Roberts*

Acknowledgments

I want to acknowledge my father, who had me swimming practically before I could walk, and encouraged my love of all sports and fitness.

To my mother Andree Look, and Susan Dey and Cher, who via their exemplification of beauty and grace instilled a true appreciation of womanhood in me.

To The Summit Publishing Group, for creating the incredible opportunity to share this information.

To Linda Shelton, my ever-enduring, unbelievably hardworking writer. There is no way I could have done this without her like-minded understanding, creativity, and enthusiasm.

To my fellow instructors, who have guided, taught, and inspired me.

To Dr. Arnold Sandlow, my wonderful chiropractor/sports medicine doctor. His treatments gave me a deeper understanding and respect for my body, which I've been able to pass on to my clients and students.

To Tobi Levine, my nutritionist, who assisted me in developing a truly healthful approach to food and eating. Her eating plan not only helped to make my body look its best, but gave my life a new freedom. I love that. Freedom!

To my dear friends, Cody, Lee, Connie, Joey, Ken, Trudy, Mitch, Nessa, and Bruce, who love and support me through all my ups and downs.

To the great staff and owners of Martin Henry Fitness Studio, where I teach and continue to learn and expand my craft and develop my programs.

To Moda Prima and Jim Torti, who supply me with outstanding workout gear.

To Ryka, who keep me in step with their excellent footwear, which I find to be the best. To all the inspirational women at the Ryka Rose Foundation, whose dedicated work toward education and aid for abused women helps thousands in desperate need throughout America today. I am so proud to be part of your incredible movement.

To Better Bodies of Los Angeles, for the use of their top-notch fitness facility for our photo shoot.

Introduction

❧

If you want something very badly, you can achieve it. It may take patience, very hard work, a real struggle, and a long time; but it can be done ... faith is a prerequisite of any understanding.
—*Margo Jones*

❧

A combination of my own painful, desperate search and a sound educational background gave birth to my own approach to fitness—real fitness. Now I have the opportunity to share it with you.

My passion for wanting to help others stems from knowing how it feels to live with a shameful sense of failure and isolation. So many people suffer, not just the "average person." In my work with the famous celebrities I've trained, I've come to see that no one is immune. No matter how rich, famous, and successful they are, Hollywood beauties also suffer from the gnawing feelings of inadequacy. Being consistently "camera-ready" isn't easy, and it's truly a mistake to think that every starlet is in picture-perfect shape all the time. Imagine the humiliation which accompanies their failures and fallacies when gaining weight becomes inevitable public punishment.

What they then do is what we all do, at some time or another . . . start again and get back on track.

My purpose in writing this book is to guide you, to help you find and keep the motivation you need to attain your goals. The solution is simpler than you think. Eat well; train smart; rest; recreate; have fun, friends, interests, and down time—it's all like a recipe. Follow it with the correct amount of all the ingredients and cook it up according to the instructions, and presto! This is the "Hollywood Cookbook of Fitness." You can choose your ingredients based upon your needs, wants, and goals, and cook yourself up an ideal body.

Notice, I said simple, not easy. There is a difference. In Dr. M. Scott Peck's bestseller *The Road Less Traveled*, his opening line is, "Life is hard." He's right. We all look for an easier, softer way. We all look for shortcuts. Every day, we're lambasted with media misinformation that preys on our vulnerable human need for instant gratification and change: quick-fix pills, creams and rubs, cellulite wraps, passive exercise programs, overnight weight-loss scams, and miracle diets. Even singer and movie star Cher was not exempt from this thinking. When we started working together, I weaned her off her meal replacement diet drinks and food bars, so she could develop a better relationship with everyday "nondiet" foods. The results were incredible; for proof, just look at her fitness video, *A New Attitude*.

So often, the instant remedy turns into the long-term nightmare. Science has shown that yo-yo dieting with quick weight loss slows the metabolism, making it easier to regain the weight back . . . and then some. My program will bring you results and it's not based on Hollywood magic, but simple, no-nonsense principles. You can and will transform your body. Just as importantly, it will improve your vitality and stamina for life, increase your strength for daily tasks, and retrain your eating habits to finally free you from endless dieting and guilt.

Yes, free you; that's a big promise. I know that changing my lifestyle to include proper exercising and eating has given me great freedom to choose a better way. Beyond my body, it has given me peace of mind, a strong spirit, and the will to stick with a program. I needed to look inside myself and find the discipline to do this. All great actors and teachers of our time will tell you that discipline, along with being in the moment, focusing, and then committing to it, is the most difficult thing to do. This is so true with exercise; it can only be done in the present . . . now, now, and right now!!!

I guarantee you an exciting and fascinating journey through this book. Along the way, you're sure to meet some truly incredible people. The most incredible one, of course, is . . . you. One more thing: Don't just read this book, use it to keep notes about yourself and your progress. There are places throughout the book for you to record notes, self-test results, personalized program workouts, etc.

ONE

Establishing Lifestyle Goals

ATTITUDE AND CHANGE
*Instead of concentrating
on why we can't do a thing,
we would be wise to change
our "yes, but …" attitude
to a more positive one.
Saying "yes" means I really
do want to change my life
for the better.*
—Liane Cordes

T he first thing I do with clients is ask them what they want to accomplish, whether it's losing weight, improving shape and tone, or simply becoming fit. But many people are reticent when it comes to being specific in putting *true* goals down on paper. In most instances, they don't really believe their desired changes will take place, so they end up protecting themselves from disappointment.

On the other end of the scale are the overly ambitious, unrealistic goal setters. Their dreams are ludicrous to the point of being absolutely unattainable. While there's nothing wrong with being a dreamer, far-out dreams likewise can set you up for disappointment and even disillusionment. The trick is to find a balance between a confident optimism and realistic standards when setting your goals.

It's time for you to take your first step toward a new life of health and fitness. Start with spending some really private, quality time with your thoughts, formulating some realistic goals true to yourself and your capabilities. A goal is something that can be *manifested;* it is a step in the right direction to direct or process change in your life. Say, for example, you would like to lose fifty pounds. Actually, you wanted to lose all of it yesterday, but now that that isn't possible, you give yourself a break and set next week for a deadline. Of course, that doesn't work in the real word, either.

Here's the straight "skinny": Your lifestyle, mainly your eating and exercise habits, needs to change in order for you to lose weight and then permanently keep off the weight. Now for that reality check—I'm talking about a good six months of commitment and then some. If you expect to lose it all in two or three weeks, you either will never start or you'll stop, because you'll feel frustrated. Here's an example of how to set up tangible, reachable goals for success:

Overall Goal (The Big Picture):

I want to lose fifty pounds within six to eight months and keep it off.

Smaller Goals (Baby Steps):

1. I will begin to exercise slowly by walking three times a week, and will strength train two times a week.
2. I will cut out all fried foods.
3. I will use the food exchange plan to monitor my overall intake.
4. I will ask my husband to do the marketing because this is when I have the habit of munching.

These goals are attainable. When you write down your goals, you need to keep looking at them—*remember* them. But make them *real!* I advise my clients to post their goals where they're most visible, usually on the fridge.

One thing I find so true with myself and my clients is that some things are easy to change, others seem impossible. It's easy to "plunge" right into some activities; with others, I need to "wade" through the process. For example, when I had long hair, then finally made the decision to cut it, I plunged right in and just about shaved my head! I didn't hold back from that one. Yet, when I knew I needed to change my eating habits, there were certain things I wasn't ready to give up: whole milk, whole cheese, fried foods, and oil. So I cut back a little bit at a time, until I could cut them out completely. I think of myself as a plunger—that's my personality, but all of us are waders about some things, and that's perfectly all right. Cher once told me, "Moderation doesn't work for me; I have to actively start a program, get into a system, and make a big change." Cher is definitely a plunger!

Here's your chance to see just how willing you are to dive headlong into the ocean, or if you need to hang out by the water's edge, sticking your toes in the water one foot at a time. These are lifestyle changes that will make the big picture much easier to achieve. You'll find that you're very willing to plunge on all or some, but only willing to wade on others. This will also clue you in about your commitment level to yourself. Look at this list periodically. You might be willing at some point to plunge where you are only now willing to wade.

Plunge or Wade . . .

THE EASIEST ATTITUDE ADJUSTMENT PROGRAM

Plunge	Wade	
❏	❏	**I am willing to subtract:** sodas. **I will substitute:** water, eight to twelve 8-ounce glasses per day.
❏	❏	**I am willing to subtract:** nonhunger eating; boredom, stress, loneliness, or anger "bingeing." **I will substitute:** a walk, cool shower or hot bath, a call to a friend, talking about my feelings, expressing my feelings.
❏	❏	**I am willing to subtract:** "blowing it off"; cutting my workout when I don't think I have the time or energy. **I will substitute:** doing it anyway . . . commit to fitting it in, even if it's not the full "perfect" session. Often when you feel tired, you'll feel better before you're halfway through!

❏ ❏ **I am willing to subtract:** being a couch potato ... Lazy habits will kill you!!!
I will substitute: being generally more active. Walk instead of drive. Find an enjoyable active hobby, such as taking the stairs or walking the dog.

❏ ❏ **I am willing to subtract:** skipping meals.
I will substitute: Breakfast! Lunch! Dinner!—healthy snacks when hungry.

❏ ❏ **I am willing to subtract:** self-neglectful habits.
I will substitute: time for self-care as my No. 1 priority. (How can you take care of anything else if your own house isn't in order?)

❏ ❏ **I am willing to subtract:** criticism and judgmental, perfectionistic self-thoughts.
I will substitute: affirming, patient, gentle, and loving encouragement toward myself and my new path.

❏ ❏ **I am willing to subtract/limit:** alcohol and cigarettes, particularly hard liquor.
I will substitute: water, nonalcoholic beverages, sugarless gum.

❏ ❏ **I am willing to subtract:** all-or-nothing thinking.
I will substitute: looking for the "gray," instead of all black or white.

❏ ❏ **I am willing to subtract:** addictive, workaholic habits.
I will substitute: permission to play aimlessly, to rest, to relax, recreate, and take time out for me.

❏ ❏ **I am willing to subtract:** the "if-onlys."
I will substitute: taking responsibility for myself with decisive action ... *now!*

❏ ❏ **I am willing to subtract:** frantic rushing.
I will substitute: prioritizing my needs and know that stressing myself out to fit it all in helps no one.

❏ ❏ **I am willing to subtract:** scaring myself with negative thinking.
I will substitute: taking a deep breath, slowing down, and replacing the thought with a more positive one.

❏ ❏ **I am willing to subtract:** blaming others for my problems.
I will substitute: looking at my part in every situation and learning about myself.

❏ ❏ **I am willing to subtract:** swallowing my feelings/letting others "walk all over me."
I will substitute: asserting myself and expressing my needs.

When setting goals for yourself, it's important to recognize the things you're willing to *plunge* on and the things that you're willing to *wade* through. More importantly, however, you must feel *comfortable with yourself* and these decisions.

∾

*If my mind can conceive it, and my heart
can believe it, I know I can achieve it.*
—*Reverend Jesse Jackson*

∾

The D.I.R.E.C.T. Approach to Lifestyle Changes and Permanent Weight Loss

Being a plunger, I like to take the direct route to get anywhere, even though that sometimes has led me straight into a brick wall. I've learned to respect my process and what I need—it can't be on anyone else's time schedule.

The D.I.R.E.C.T. approach to goal setting will help you establish permanent lifestyle changes. Think of the areas in your life that you want to work on, then follow this formula:

Define your needs
Increase activity
Reconstruct dietary habits
Establish support
Commit to your goals
Time . . . be patient

When you have a quiet moment, find a sitting place alone that feels comfortable to you. Have paper and pen handy; you're going to write some goals based on the D.I.R.E.C.T. method. Follow these guidelines to help you make your goals more real:

1. State your goals in the form of "I." This makes them personal because they belong to you.

2. Establish the big picture and the baby steps to get you there.

3. Give yourself a time frame, so you know what you want to accomplish within it.

4. If you need support, determine who or what will supply it for you.

5. Put these where you can see them and read them every day. To make goals real is to make them believable to yourself.

My Goals

Date today: _____

1. The Big Picture: **I** _____

_____

2. Baby Steps: **I will**

　　1. _____

　　2. _____

　　3. _____

　　4. _____

　　5. _____

3. Time frame:

　　1. Big Picture _____

　　2. Baby steps _____

4. I need support from _____

_____

Achieving Positive Self-Change

The first step in making positive self-change is to look at the relationship that you have with yourself—your self-concept. Our motivation to succeed, whether it be physical or mental, comes from within us. Developing a healthy self-concept will lead to positive thoughts and positive results. For example, if you can say to yourself, "I love having exercise in my life, I love to move," your attitude about it will be "I feel great!" Your response to exercise will then be "I'm ready for more, I'm ready to be active," which leads to a very positive feeling about keeping exercise in your life. Always remember, *you* get to choose what you do.

In the following "Goal-Tending" section, you get a self-inventory guide to assist you in formulating a health-and-fitness plan suited to self-change.

Goal-Tending

- Communicate honestly with yourself. Withholding truth from yourself could seriously compromise your progress.

- Be clear about what you want from this program, what you want from yourself, and how much of your time and energy you're willing to commit to it.

- Choose the methods best suited to who you are, your needs, your lifestyle, and how you "operate in your life."

- Be realistic about what you expect to look like . . . your genetics will influence where you hold your body fat, your general body shape, limb length, and hip width.

- How quickly you get results will depend upon your level of commitment, how much you are willing to do, and how precisely you stick to it.

- It's okay to go at your own pace. If weight loss is your goal, I recommend losing no more than two pounds per week.

- Be patient, flexible, and gentle with yourself. You're sure to slip, slide, and wander . . . just keep recommitting. Have faith in the process. It is a process, and within that process you will discover a new body and perhaps even a new person within that body.

- Consistency rather than perfection is your greatest friend. Throwing the baby out with the bathwater is going to leave you with nothing.

- Create support with your family, work peers, and social groups. Don't be afraid to communicate your needs and get group back-up from them: I can't . . . we can! You might even motivate a few others along the way.

- Be willing to let go of whatever it is you use to justify your overeating habits. Rigorous honesty is called for here—your dishonesty could be those few extra inches round your waistline.

A Realistic Look at Cutting the Food Chain

Contrary to what advertisers would have us believe, food is *not* a form of entertainment, stress release, or relaxation. It is not your lover, friend, or even your enemy. It is necessary physical nourishment.

A STEP-BY-STEP SHORTCUT TO GET GOING NOW . . .
1. **Wholesome** . . . Eat natural, unprocessed, or lightly processed food. Choose the whole food whenever possible, such as brown rice rather than white, whole grain instead of white bread, baked potato with the skin on rather than potato chips, corn on the cob rather than corn chips, whole apples rather than the juice.

2. **Moderate** . . . Anything in moderation, even ice cream, hot dogs, etc., will fit into the big picture of an otherwise low-fat, healthy diet. Too much of anything will eventually tip the scale to add up

to a junk-food diet. Try balancing it out by making sure the rest of your food choices are wholesome and healthy.

3. **Variety** . . . is the spice of life. There is no single magical food which will provide all your nutritional answers. We need to consume a wide variety of grains, fruits, vegetables, meats, low-fat dairy products, and unsaturated fats. Not only will your diet be balanced, it also will never become boring.

4. **Choice** . . . If something in my program doesn't suit you, find an option that does! There are plenty of choices available. It's important to find a path you can most comfortably follow. Tailor it to yourself. I know this so clearly from the many diverse personality types I've worked with. The food program I gave to Kirstie Alley is completely different from the one that I created for Susan Dey, and different again from the program for Cher or even Faye Dunaway.

5. **Regular** . . . Skipping meals is a giant no-no!! This is true no matter what is going on or how busy you might think you are. If you think you are too busy to slow down enough to nourish yourself, then perhaps you need to examine your priorities. After all, you would never be too busy to stop to get gas for your fuel tank if it were empty. Don't you think it's strange that we often take better care of our cars than we do our bodies?

You Are the Priority

The biggest stumbling block I see with clients is their inability to regard themselves, their needs, and wants as a priority. Guilt takes over as the leading character. Women, who naturally take on the family nurturer's role, have a particularly difficult time setting aside even a half hour for private time, whether it be for exercise or a much-needed nap. *Allowing* yourself to be a priority as well as prioritizing your goals—while giving yourself a little time without guilt—can be the key to positive self-growth and self-change.

Slipping and Sliding

Backsliding is part of human nature. We wouldn't be human if we didn't stray. In my experience with slipping (I've slipped, tripped, stumbled, and fallen more than you would ever believe), the most valuable lesson I've learned is to be gentle, quick to forgive, and unconditionally loving with myself. I swear that if loving myself were contingent on my being able to achieve something right away, I'd still be where I was years ago, filled with self-loathing and acting out those feelings.

Learning to be human and accepting my human fallibility seems my most challenging and ongoing life lesson. Yet, it is my most rewarding. As I have learned to love and accept myself as imperfect, I've learned to love and accept the people in my life unconditionally, which in turn has given me the opportunity to establish truly nurturing and mutually loving relationships.

Your dreams come true when you act to turn them into realities.
—Heart Warmers

Notes

Notes

Notes

Notes

TWO

Self-Assessment

SELF
*To be what we are,
and to become what
we are capable of
is the only end in life.*
—Robert L. Stevenson

One of the first things I do with a new client is ask what his or her immediate and long-term goals are. Typically, getting in better shape and losing a few pounds top the list. Before I can prescribe a personalized program, I need to find out what kind of shape my client is in.

You need to know your starting point before you can plan and track successful progress. Like planning a battle, you need to know where you are in relation to the "enemy." That's why I'm going to guide you through a number of easy self-assessments so you take a nonjudgmental look at yourself. These assessments are not about right and wrong, or good and bad; they are merely a measuring stick which you can use to gain perspective on where you are and where you need to go. Notice I said measuring stick, not whipping stick . . . I mean it, too! This is not an excuse to beat up yourself. Consider it more of a chance to step out into the light and see what's there. Look in the mirror and observe yourself, even if it might be a painfully hard task. But give yourself permission to move forward because this is the biggest "baby step" you'll ever take!

Six-Step Reflective Inventory

This inventory will provide some genuine information about yourself and give you specific guidance to setting some realistic, nonthreatening goals. Again, this activity is *not* a flogging session if you don't believe you measure up perfectly to society's dictates. It's about recognition, acceptance, and making an attitude shift; you just need to be willing. This will help you recognize the effect that culture has had on your self-image, especially if you have a poor one.

Society is the culprit. We are being told over and over that in order to be loved and accepted, we have to be a perfect, ideal, feminine size. I *know*. I spent so many years alternately rebelling (getting fat and saying I didn't care anyway) or punishing myself into some form of conformity (by creating a body that I could maintain only with starvation). Basically, what I wanted was a different body type, not an improvement of the old one. I wanted to trade in for a petite, willowy, Scarlett O'Hara figure with an eighteen-inch waist, voluptuous breasts, delicate arms, and thin legs. Instead, I was five-foot-ten, broad shouldered, flat chested, narrow hipped, boyish looking, muscular, and athletic. I hated it; not only did I have huge hands and feet, I was constantly being mistaken as my mother's other son!

Before I realized it, I was desperate for something I could never have. I've since learned to choose healthier role models—women with similar genetics, bone structures, and body types. The idea isn't trying to be someone you're not; it's making the best of what you have.

You must take an honest look at your body; not the way you *believe* you look, but the way you *actually* look. The following six steps will help you inventory the things that you really like about your body, as well as the things that you'd like to change. Spend some time with this process and get to know yourself. Record your observations on the Reflective Inventory Guide at the end of this chapter. To have a positive, nurturing, self-accepting relationship with yourself is first and foremost; it's the real reward far beyond the quest for perfection.

1. Make sure you have at least ten minutes of uninterrupted time for yourself.

2. You'll need a private, quiet, well-lit room with a full-length mirror.

3. Remove your clothing so you can get a good look at yourself.

4. Study your body first from the front, then from each side, and finally, with a hand mirror, look at your backside. Observe yourself; notice your body structure; see if anything looks out of proportion; observe how you stand and carry yourself, and if you need to tone your muscles.

5. Be rigorously honest; not viciously brutal . . . make notes to yourself as if you are speaking to your closest friend.

6. Be realistic. Try not to overdramatize how "awful" you think you might look. Remember, you're about to start a program which will give you results!

These are merely suggestions; you don't have to do it this way. Whichever way you do it, however, be honest and gentle. I included this inventory guide because for so many years I used the mirror as a form of self-punishment. I somehow felt that if I continued to hate myself as much as I did, I could force myself to both not eat and yet work out hard. I now know that this "technique" only served to continue my self-destructive habits of yo-yo dieting and binge-purge behavior with food and exercise.

Redefining Your Mirror Image

Dismiss your internal, judgmental committee; you know, those discerning, hateful voices that tell you that your legs aren't long enough, your body isn't curvy or busty enough, or that you're fat. You need to really take a true personal inventory. If you can be the final judge of what you look like rather than rely on the "yeah, but" committee in your head or society, you can probably paint a true, healthy picture of who you are.

Get back in front of the mirror, have your inventory guide handy, grab a pen and a tape measure, and let's assess a few things.

A. First, let's be honest. While we all have a "body wish list," there's some things we can't change. If you have "short legs," there isn't an exercise in the world that can lengthen them, but we can change leg shape through exercise and healthy eating.

Use the inventory guide to jot down some notes. You'll be able to look at this periodically and see the progress you've made, physically as well as mentally. Look again at yourself from the front, from the sides, and from the rear. Really *look* at your body from an objective point of view. Notice where your body curves and where it indents. Observe if your shoulders are narrower or broader than your hips, or if they round forward. Remember, no bashing, just looking. Jot down the things that you: (1) really like—that make you attractive to yourself; (2) accept or acknowledge, or inherited (such as your dad's hands) that can't be changed; and (3) don't like, yet you know you can change.

Make sure you include positive things about yourself; this is the hard part, because it's easier to criticize. I think I have really pretty ankles and I've always liked them. When I was at my heaviest, and felt really bad about everything, I'd look at my ankles and tell myself how nice they were so that I could feel positive about something. We all need to be able to do this. It's also important that you're realistic about the hereditary and genetic traits that make you unique to your family. Most people can find a distinct resemblance to other family members. Make sure you are not finding fault with yourself because of your feelings about the person you most resemble. Once you can begin to accept the things you can't change, it will be easier to strive for the things that you can change.

B. Next, let's try and determine your body type and frame size. This is important, because the exercises you'll be choosing in chapter 7 for program design will partially be determined by what it is you want to accomplish. Different exercises work best for certain body types, but we'll be talking about that later.

The most widely used method to determine body type is somato-typing, which groups bodies into three main types: (1) endomorph, (2) mesomorph, and (3) ectomorph. Look in the mirror again.

1. If you have a softer, rounded, or hourglass shape, you are proba-bly an endomorph. Endomorphs classically carry their body weight more around the abdomen and hips, have narrow shoul-ders, larger breasts, broader hips and buttocks, and heavier thighs, often giving the appearance of an overloaded bottom half. Endomorphs gain fat easily, but have a tough time gaining mus-cle. With the right program, however, endomorphs respond well to a solid weight-training program that targets the large muscle groups to pare down the hips and thighs, while building shoul-ders and back to create a more symmetrical look. If you're a true endomorph, you may never see those deep cuts in your muscles, but you can expect an overall well-toned physique.

2. If you are more muscular, athletic looking, heavier boned, and more rectangular, you are a mesomorph. Mesomorphs tend to be fairly symmetrical, so when they gain weight, they gain it propor-tionately, though mesomorphs typically don't gain fat easily. Muscle mass does comes easy and a balanced weight-training program is the perfect avenue for defining and toning.

3. If you have a more slender shape and a more frail body structure with long limbs, nondefinitive breasts and hips, you are an ecto-morph. That makes you one of the "natural" skinnies envied by many. Ectomorphs are less inclined to gain fat or muscle, but they can become flabby without exercise. If you're an ectomorph, your body will respond well to a toning program using lighter weights.

Although you are probably described as one of these three body types, you more likely are a combination or a variation of them. Cher, for example, is a classic endomorph who is in great shape. She has narrow shoulders, long limbs, but pear-shaped hips and thighs. We worked really hard on her entire body to improve her symmetry and gain muscle. On the other hand, Kirstie Alley was a combination of a mesomorph and endomorph. Although she has a tendency to gain weight easily, she also gained muscle easily. While working together, we had to concentrate on a program that emphasized muscular endurance, while using light weights and a high volume of repetitions.

These descriptions will give you a general genetic guideline because you will live forever with your body type. However, this is just part of it. As I've described, each body type responds well to certain programs. Mark down which body type you think you are, add any appropriate notes, and then let's move on.

Oops, wait a minute; don't put your clothes on yet. Let's do one more thing. Remember, today is a starting point, so you need all the data—much like a scientist—so you can chart your continued progress.

Make sure that you weigh yourself today. But don't let the power of the scale rule you. Weigh in only once a week. Next, it's time to take your measurements. Even if you can pinch more than an inch and you know you need to lose weight, monitoring these circumference changes while you're in transition provides a simple guideline to let you see how your body responds to your program. You'll need a cloth measuring tape to do this. Measure yourself at the sites listed below. Hold the tape gently without slack, but not so tight that your skin wrinkles:

1. **Chest:** around your back and across nipple level

2. **Waist:** at the narrowest part of your torso, where it indents to form your waist

3. **Hips:** around your buttocks at the roundest or widest part

4. **Thigh:** just below the fold of your buttocks

5. **Lower thigh:** midway between your hips and knees

6. **Knee:** just above the top of your knee

7. **Calf:** at the largest spot between knee and ankle

8. **Upper arm:** midway between shoulder and elbow

9. **Forearm:** largest part with arm extended, palm forward

After today, put your mirror inventory away until you've been on your new program at least four to seven weeks. One more thing—take pride in having taken the time to get to know yourself; it took a lot of courage. Remember the rhyme, "Mirror, mirror on the wall, whose the fairest of them all?" Perhaps today, or soon, you'll discover it's you.

Fat Chance

These are just numbers, but they *do* represent you. Now you know from determining your body type and taking your measurements where most of your fat lies or where your tendency to gain fat is. If you carry fat around your middle, you have what is commonly referred to as an "apple" shape; if you carry your fat in hips and thighs and you're narrow on top, this is called a "pear" shape.

Where body fat accumulates isn't just a cosmetic issue, it's important to health. Medical practitioners agree that too much fat can be hazardous to your health. Studies have shown if you are an apple shape, there is a higher risk for heart disease, diabetes, or other metabolic disorders. To determine your level of risk when it comes to fat and your health, use your waist/hip ratio. Divide your waist measurement by your hip measurement. If you're a woman with a ratio greater than .85, or .95 if you're a man, then you would be considered a higher risk.

Other factors that will help you determine this, along with your fat-distribution risk, are blood pressure, and cholesterol and triglyceride levels. Compare them with standard norms. This doesn't mean you *will* have heart problems. Remember, you're in the driver's seat: A proper exercise program and diet will give you control.

Body-Fat Basics

You have a lot of facts and figures about yourself that will change as you exercise. Did you notice that I haven't given you any standard comparison charts so you can see if you're "normal"? Most of the traditional height/weight charts are inaccurate when it comes to determining how much you should weigh. If you have a lot of muscle mass and low body fat, you'll weigh more, which could make you "fat" on the chart, but underfat in reality.

The Body Mass Index (BMI) is an easy and quick way to determine a more healthy weight for you; it's certainly better than comparing yourself to unreasonable norms. Place one end of a ruler on your exact height on the right column of the following chart and the other end on your exact weight on the left column. Where the ruler crosses in the middle is your BMI.

If you're a woman and your BMI falls between 19 and 24 (up to 26 if you're more than thirty-five years old or male), that's acceptable and probably a reasonably good body weight for you. If you're above these numbers, keep the right end of the ruler constant, and move the other end of the ruler so the middle settles somewhere around 21 or 22. Your weight will show on the left side of the ruler. Remember, these numbers are only an estimate to give you some guidelines.

A factor more important than your weight or hip size is how much of the weight is actually fat and how much is what we call lean body mass (consisting of your bones, muscles, organs, and tissues). By referring to how much *fat* you have rather than your *weight* will give you a more realistic assessment, particularly because body type can be deceiving. A person who "looks" thin can have less fat subcutaneously (below the level of the skin), but actually have a high percentage of fat around organs and between muscles. Knowing your lean body

BMI Index Chart

(Source: G. A. Bray, "Definitions, Measurements and Classification of the Syndromes of Obesity," International Journal of Obesity, John Libbey and Company, 1978.)

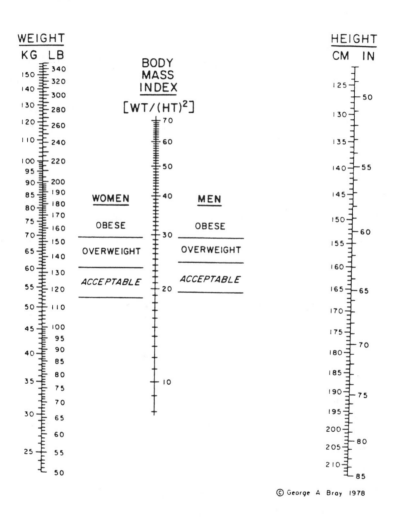

© George A. Bray 1978

mass/fat ratio will help you determine a healthy and optimal weight, as well as plan a sound diet and exercise attack.

To determine your body-fat percentage, place one end of your trusty ruler on your height on the right column of the following chart and the other end on your hip measurement in the left column. Where the ruler crosses in the center is your body-fat percentage. This is an estimated number with a 3-5 percent margin of error, so you could be a little more or a little less. If you are a woman and between 19 and 24 percent, that's great! For men, these numbers are a little lower—15-18 percent.

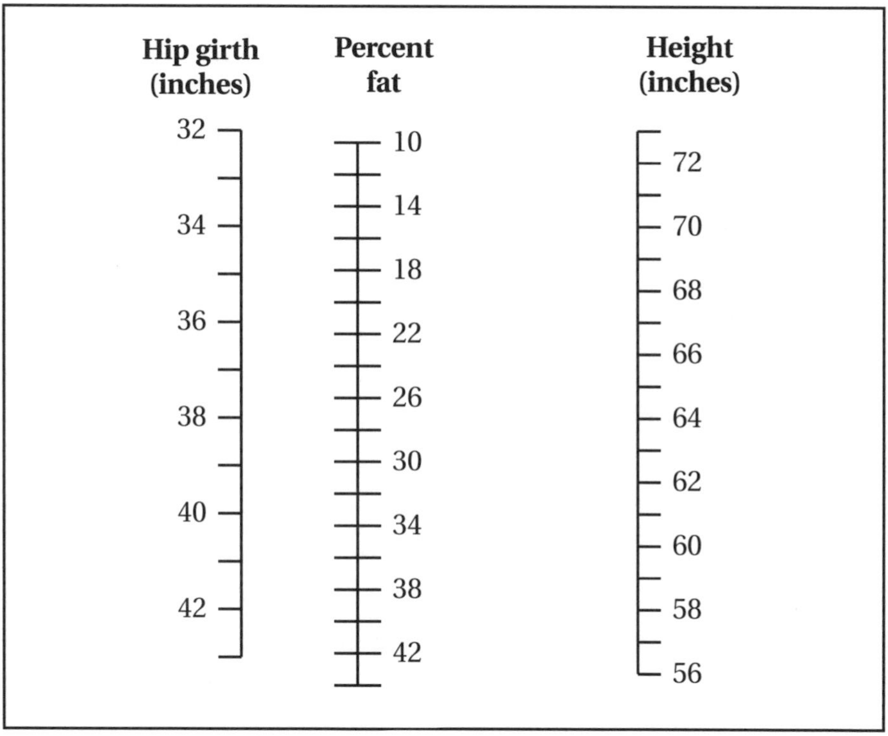

Hip girth (inches)	Percent fat	Height (inches)
32	10	72
34	14	70
	18	68
36	22	66
38	26	64
	30	62
40	34	60
42	38	58
	42	56

To determine your lean body mass (LBM)/fat ratio, use the following formula:

Example: Mary, age 32

	Body weight		135
x	% fat	x	.27
	————————		————————
=	pounds of fat		37 pounds of fat
	Your body weight		135
-	pounds of fat	-	37
	————————		————————
=	lean body mass		98

Most of us fluctuate a little in weight; that's normal. Instead of constantly striving to stay at a perfect, ideal number, you want to stay within a healthy range. Based on body-fat percentages, a healthy LBM for women is between .81 and .76 (19-24 percent fat). If you're a man, this would be .85 and .82. Divide your lean body mass by these numbers, according to your sex.

If we use our example woman, the equation would look like this:

$98 \div .81 = 121$ pounds

$98 \div .76 = 129$ pounds

Based on these calculations, Mary needs to lose between six and fourteen pounds of fat to be at her ideal weight. At the most, this should take only three to four months. The important thing to remember is we're talking about losing *fat*, not lean body mass; you don't want to lose muscle. The easiest way to do this is to add exercise to your life.

Health Beyond the Perfect Body

Weighing Your Risk

When I ask my new clients why they want to exercise, they rarely answer, "To make me healthy and increase my longevity." They have the same reason you do for reading this book; you want to get your body together, *now*. Don't get me wrong, that's fine—it's what got me started initially. But under the guise of body reform, your health will also improve.

You've heard over and over again that exercise is beneficial to your health. Whittling down your waistline will do more than diminish fat; it reduces "fat disease." Doctors are now taking a no-nonsense, assertive approach in recommending exercise to protect against heart disease and its associated illnesses such as obesity, diabetes, and hypertension. Some of these factors, like a sedentary lifestyle, can be controlled through your own determination to stick to diet and exercise. Some other factors, such as family history, are uncontrollable factors in our lives. The important thing is, if you recognize and acknowledge them, you then can deal effectively. It might be that you'll have to make definitive, bold changes in your life, but these changes will give you *your life*.

∾

ACTION
Acceptance is not submission; it is acknowledgment of the facts of a situation, then deciding what you're going to do about it.
—Kathleen Casey Theisen

∾

Your body is a complex mechanism, just like a well-tuned automobile. When something is out of sync, a flashing light indicates that something is wrong. We often don't pay attention to our body's signals, and some of them are not as obvious. When it comes to our bodies, "ignorance is risk"!

The following self-assessments will help you identify lifestyle habits as well as establish exercise guidelines: how much to start with, how long to do them, and how hard you should work. Again, this is not about being right or wrong. If you haven't exercised in a while, or have never exercised, you already should know you need to start off slowly.

The good news is that within a month or two, these numbers will change. Jot down your scores on your inventory guide and then retest about every eight to twelve weeks. This initial look at yourself will help you chart progress and attain your future goals.

Risk Factor Profile

This risk factor questionnaire was adapted from the RISKO American Heart Association profile to identify potential heart risk. Answer each question, totaling your score for each category. Then add your scores together to interpret your risk.

A. Uncontrollable Factors

1. **Age**

Under 30	0	Score_____
30-44	1	
45-54	2	
55-64	4	
Over 65	6	

2. **Sex**

Female	0	Score_____
Male	5	

3. **Family history of heart disease (parents, siblings, uncles, and aunts)**

None	0	Score_____
1 or 2	1	
2 or more	3	
Younger than 40, add 4 points.		

4. **Diabetes**

Absent	0	Score_____
Present	3	

   PART A Subtotal_____

B. Controllable Factors

5. Stress

Low	0	Score_____
Moderate	2	
High	4	

6. Regular exercise

Very Active	0	Score_____
Moderate	1	
Little	2	
Sedentary	4	

7. Smoking

Never	0	Score_____
Cigar or Pipe	1	
Cigarettes:		
None for at least		
8 years or more	0	
None for 3-8 years	1	
In the past 3 years:		
Less than 1/2 pack per day	4	
Up to 1 pack per day	6	
1-2 packs per day	8	

8. Weight

Less than 15 pounds over	0	Score_____
15-30 pounds over	1	
More than 30 pounds over	2	

PART B Subtotal_____

C. Medical Data

9. **Total cholesterol**

Under 190	0	Score_____
190-209	1	
210-219	2	
220-239	4	
240-259	6	
Over 260	8	

10. **HDL cholesterol**

Over 50	0	Score_____
45-49	2	
35-44	4	
25-34	6	
Below 25	8	

11. **Triglycerides**

Below 150	0	Score_____
151-200	1	
Over 200	2	

12. **Blood Pressure**

Below 140/85	0	Score_____
Below 150/90	1	
Below 160-95	2	
Below 170/100	4	
Below 175/105	6	
Higher reading	8	

PART C Subtotal_____

Grand Total Score_____

Risk score interpretation:

Below 12	Low risk
13-26	Modest risk
27-37	Moderate risk
Above 38	High risk

If medical data is not available, use the following scale:

Below 10	Low risk
11-15	Modest risk
16-21	Moderate risk
Above 22	High risk

You might want to consult your doctor before starting any new exercise program, particularly if you need to clean up unhealthy habits. The American College of Sports Medicine recommends that you have a physician's clearance prior to exercising if you (1) are a female over fifty or male over forty; and/or (2) have any known cardiopulmonary or metabolic disease; or (3) have two or more of the aforementioned risk factors present.

After taking this profile, weigh your risks. Are they controllable or uncontrollable? Remember, too, that risk is relative. Could you de-stress a little, change your eating habits, and add exercise to your life—knowing it could improve or save your life? Probably. Since many of these risk factors are controllable, you can do something about it.

On the Far Side of Fat Is Fit

Is there no happy medium between being fit and fat? Well, unfortunately, you can't get fit overnight, particularly if you've been on the couch, chowing down Doritos. But there is a continuum that takes us from Point A to Point B, and beyond. We just need a starting point. But first, let's look at the components that make up fitness.

1. Aerobic conditioning is the capacity of cardiovascular and respiratory systems to process oxygen so the body can sustain moderate to vigorous exercise for a long period of time. A variety of activities, such as walking, running, biking, swimming, roller blading, rowing, stepping, or aerobic dance exercise can improve the condition of your heart and lungs.

2. Muscular strength is the ability of your muscles to exert maximal force against a resistance for a single repetition. Activities such as weight training will strengthen muscles as well as joints and connective tissue so that you can perform daily tasks more easily with reduced risk of injury.

3. Muscular endurance is the ability of your muscles to exert sub-maximal force during an extended period of time (or hold a static contraction), like when you do a lot of repetitions with a light-weight resistance. When you prolong exercise time, you are also improving the endurance of your heart muscle.

4. Flexibility is the ability of your muscles to lengthen beyond their normal resting length and increase the available range of motion of your joints.

We're going to assess each of these components separately. Follow the directions carefully for each quiz, then mark your scores on your inventory guide, so that you can come back to it later.

Cardiovascular Assessment

To test your cardiovascular system, you need to know how to take your heart rate and how to figure your training heart-rate range. To find your pulse, wrap four fingers around the outside of your wrist, closest to your thumb. Don't panic, one of your fingers *will* find a pulse.

You'll be using this heart-rate monitoring system for a variety of things. First, take your pulse at your wrist in the morning for three mornings in a row, before you get out of bed and before the alarm rings. Count your pulse for sixty seconds, then take an average over the three days. This is your resting heart rate. It's important, because a lower resting heart rate usually indicates a higher level of fitness. As you get in better shape, and continue to check this number every few months or so, you'll notice it will drop.

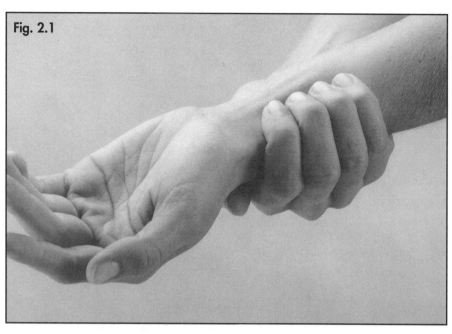

Fig. 2.1

Your resting pulse also helps determine what your training heart-rate range should be. Your training heart-rate range is the most efficient and safe zone within which you should work out and train your heart. The range that is most beneficial is 55 percent to 85 percent of your estimated maximum heart rate. You don't want to work out at maximal levels—it's too intense and you'd only be able to sustain this for a very short time. Therefore, work out at a percentage of this number. Use this formula to find your optimal personal range:

	220
-	your age
———————	
=	Estimated maximum heart rate (MHR)

THEN	Estimated MHR
-	your resting pulse
———————	
=	HR reserve

THEN   HR reserve

x   .55

_____

+   your resting pulse

_____

=   lower end of training heart-rate range

Then do the same by multiplying your heart-rate reserve by .85 to find the high end of your range.

Here's an example: Mary is 30 and has a resting pulse of 70

	220	
-	30	
___	___	___
=	190	
-	70	
___	___	___
=	120 (HRR)	120 (HRR)
x	.55	x .85
___	___	___
=	66 + 70	102 + 70
___	___	___
=	136 (low end of THRR)	172 (high end of THRR)

When Mary exercises aerobically, she wants to stay between 136 and 172. We'll talk more about heart rate in chapter 4.

To assess your cardiovascular fitness, perform either or both of the following tests. At the end of each test, you'll be taking your pulse rate at your wrist. This is called your recovery rate. The better shape you're in, the faster your heart rate will return to pre-exercise heart rates. A lowered recovery rate is a reliable sign of improved cardiovascular fitness.

Three-Minute Step Test

1. Use a step or bench that is eight inches high.

2. Step up, up, down, down, completing 24 step-ups every 60 seconds. This is approximately 96 beats per minute if you want to use music or a metronome.

3. Step for three minutes, changing which leg you're stepping up with first every minute.

4. Once you begin, keep stepping until exactly three minutes have passed.

5. At three minutes, watch your second hand and exactly 30 seconds after stopping, take your pulse for 30 seconds.

6. Compare your recovery heart rate for your age with the following chart.

7. Record your score on your inventory profile so that you can compare it next time you take this test.

Step Test Scores
Based on 30-second recovery heart rate*

(Adapted and based on information by J. J. Montoye, "Physical Activity and Health: An Epidemiologic Study of an Entire Community," Englewood Cliffs, New Jersey: Prentice-Hall, 1975.)

CLASSIFICATION	AGE			
	20-29	**30-39**	**40-49**	**50+**
WOMEN				
Excellent	39-42	39-42	41-43	41-44
Good	43-44	43-45	44-45	45-47
Average	45-46	46-47	46-47	48-49
Fair	47-52	48-53	48-54	50-55
Poor	53-66	54-66	55-67	56-66
MEN				
Excellent	34-36	35-38	37-39	37-40
Good	37-40	39-41	40-42	41-43
Average	41-42	42-43	43-44	44-45
Fair	43-47	44-47	45-49	46-49
Poor	48-59	48-59	50-60	50-62

* Thirty-second heart rate is counted beginning thirty seconds after exercise stops.

Rockport Fitness Walking Test

(A. Kasiwa and J. Rippe, Rockport Fitness Walking for Women, *New York: Putnam Publishing Group, 1987. Copyright 1987 by the Rockport Company.)*

1. Measure a mile to walk that is flat. (Most high school tracks are a quarter-mile long. Make sure that your walk is exactly one mile.
2. Take a watch with a second hand with you and walk the measured mile briskly at a steady pace.

3. At the end of the distance, immediately take your pulse rate at your wrist for ten seconds, then multiply that number by six to determine your one-minute working heart rate.

4. Note how long it took you to walk the mile. Record your heart rate and walking time on your inventory profile.

5. To determine your cardiovascular fitness level, compare your score with the profiles shown here for your age.

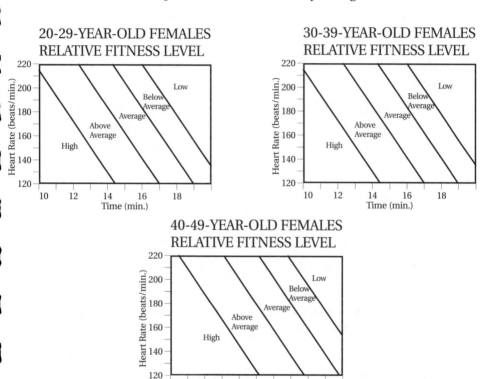

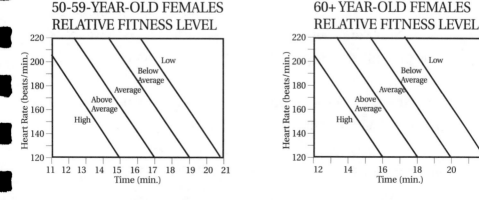

The bottom line represents your time; the line on the left represents your heart rate. The spot where these lines cross represents your fitness level. This shows the relative fitness level for others of your age group as adapted from established fitness norms set by the American Heart Association.

Strength and Endurance Assessment

Increasing muscular strength and improving endurance are crucial parts of fitness. This will keep your bones strong, and your muscles balanced and well toned, thus helping prevent injury—particularly as you get older. Developing overall strength and endurance will increase your lean body mass, which can increase your metabolism and have a definite, positive effect on body fat control. I can't begin to tell you how important it is to include exercises for strength; I feel very "strongly" about this! Now, let's get started with the strength and endurance assessment exercises!

Sit-up Crunch:

For the abdominals. All you need for this one is a stopwatch and a mat if you have hard floors. *(For proper technique, refer to setup and action photos for abdominal curls in chapter 10.)*

1. Lie on your back with your knees bent and feet flat on the floor about eighteen inches away from your buttocks.

2. Place hands behind head, but not clasped, elbows open.

3. To perform a single crunch, curl your head, neck, and shoulders upward until your shoulder blades clear the floor, then lower back to the ground, touching the floor with your shoulders.

4. Count the number of sit-up crunches that you can do in one minute and record your score on your inventory profile.

5. Compare your scores for your age with the following chart.

Sit-up Crunch Norms for One Minute

(Fitness Theory and Practice, *editor Peg Jordan, R.N., Aerobics and Fitness Association of America and Reebok University Press Publishers, 1993.*)

CLASSIFICATION			AGE		
	20-29	30-39	40-49	50-59	60+
WOMEN					
Excellent	53-66	48-59	41-50	35-43	29-36
Good	42-52	37-37	32-40	27-34	23-28
Average	30-42	25-36	22-31	17-26	15-22
Fair	16-29	13-24	12-21	8-16	6-14
Poor	0-15	0-12	0-11	0-7	0-5
MEN					
Excellent	58-71	53-64	47-57	41-50	35-43
Good	47-47	41-52	37-46	32-40	28-34
Average	35-46	28-40	26-36	22-31	19-27
Fair	20-34	14-27	14-25	12-21	10-18
Poor	0-19	0-13	0-13	0-11	0-9

Push-up:

For the chest, rear arms, and shoulders. All you need is a mat if you are going to do the modified push-up. (*For proper technique, refer to setup and action photos for push-ups in chapter 9.*)

1. Use either the full push-up position with hands just in front of shoulders and feet extended behind you or the modified position with knees just behind hips. For either position, your body should be straight with abdominals contracted.

2. Bend your elbows and lower your body until your chest almost touches the floor, then straighten arms and push back up to starting position without locking your elbows.

3. Your chest should come within three inches of the floor each time for the repetition to count.

4. Do as many push-ups with good form that you can until you can't do any more.

5. Write your score on your inventory profile.

6. Compare your score for your age with the following chart.

Push-up Norms

(Personal Trainer Manual: The Resource for Fitness Instructors,
American Council on Exercise, 1991.)

Classification	Age				
	20-29	30-39	40-49	50-59	60+
WOMEN (modified position)					
Excellent	33+	34+	28+	23+	21+
Good	23-32	22-33	18-27	15-22	13-20
Minimum	12-22	10-21	8-17	7-14	5-12
Below					
minimum	1-11	0-9	0-7	0-6	0-4
Poor	0	0	0	0	0
MEN (standard position)					
Excellent	43+	37+	31+	28+	27+
Good	30-42	25-36	21-30	18-27	17-26
Minimum	17-29	13-24	11-20	9-17	6-16
Below					
minimum	4-16	2-12	1-10	0-8	0-5
Poor	3	1	0	0	0

Flexibility Assessment

Having flexible, supple muscles decreases the risk of injury, particularly where the lower back is concerned. When your hamstrings are tight, they have the tendency to pull your spine out of its neutral alignment, sometimes causing muscle imbalance as well as pain. Flexibility is joint specific; that means each joint has its own level of range of motion. This can differ between upper and lower body joints, as well as on right and left sides of your body. These two tests pinpoint tight, inflexible shoulder and hip joints, and indicate that you definitely should add some extra stretching for these muscles to your new program.

Sit and Reach:

For lower back and hamstrings. You'll need a ruler for this.

1. Take your shoes off so that you are in socks or are barefoot.

2. Sit on the floor with your legs straight in front of you, feet flexed. (See Fig. 2.2)

3. Place a ruler between your feet, and hold it tightly between your big toes so that it rests on the front of your shins with the end marked "0" toward you.

4. Place one hand on top of the other with fingertips aligned. Keep your legs straight, but not locked, and stretch forward with arms straight toward or past your toes—without bouncing. (See Fig. 2.3)

5. Note on the ruler how far you have stretched. Return to starting position and repeat at least two more times; each time, try to stretch a little farther.

6. Do this stretch gently and cautiously, especially if your lower back and hamstrings are naturally tight.

7. Note the score of the greatest distance that you stretched on your inventory guide.

8. Each month you'll check your score to see how far you've stretched, and compare with your previous score. Here are some general guidelines:

Poor:	if you can only reach your knees or shins
Average:	if you can reach your ankles
Good:	if you can reach your toes
Excellent:	if you can reach past your toes

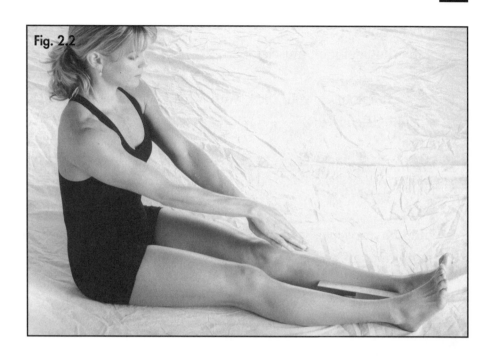

Fig. 2.2

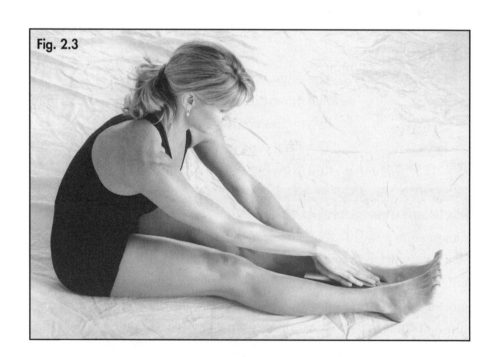

Fig. 2.3

Shoulder flexibility:

For the shoulder joint muscles.

1. Lie on the floor on your back, with arms by your sides and legs straight. (See Fig. 2.4)

2. Contract your abdominals so your lower back is as close to the floor as possible.

3. Lift both arms overhead, placing hands on the floor so your fingertips touch.(See Fig. 2.5)

4. Try to get the back of your shoulders against the floor with your lower back and fingers still on the floor.

5. Compare your flexibility with the following chart.

Evaluation of Shoulder Flexibility

Flexibility	Characteristics
MEN AND WOMEN	
Good	The fingertips can touch.
Fair	The fingertips are not touching, but are less than two inches apart.
Poor	The fingertips are more than two inches apart and arms are not on the floor.

Posture Assessment

Your posture is the last thing to assess, but it certainly isn't the least important. How you stand and hold yourself not only indicates muscle support and balance, but sometimes also reflects your feelings toward others and yourself. When you're having a bad day, you feel like slouching, slinking off into a corner, and making yourself smaller. Your shoulders get round,

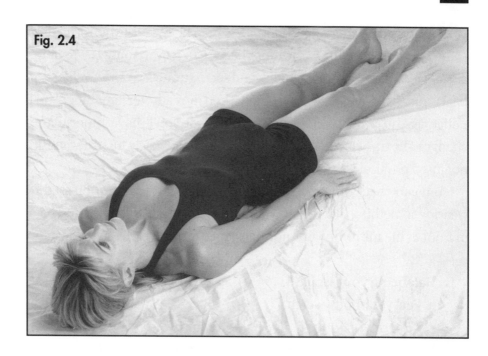

Fig. 2.4

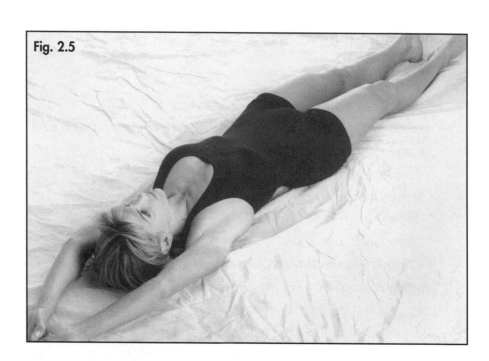

Fig. 2.5

your head hangs, and your abdominals pooch, because you really don't want to face the world. On the other hand, when everything is wonderful and life feels grand, you stand taller and seem stronger; your shoulders are back, and head and chest are lifted—you're ready for anything. You'll notice as you progress in your program that you'll have more than a change of heart. Self-esteem and posture are very closely intermeshed; it's not just a physical issue.

You can check your posture at any time when you're undressed or wearing something that reveals your body. When you're ready, stand back in front of the mirror in your normal stance and observe the following:

1. **Balancing your weight:**
   a. Feel your body weight.
   Is it forward on the balls of your feet or back on your heels?
   b. Feel where your weight is balanced from side to side.
   Are you standing on one leg more than the other?
   ++ To be balanced, you should be able to lift your toes or raise your heels without your weight balance changing.

2. **Face the mirror:**
   a. Look at your feet.
   Do they toe in or toe out?
   Do you roll your ankles inward or outward?
   ++Your feet should point straight ahead, or slightly out in a comfortable stance, with ankles straight.
   b. Look at your knees.
   Are you knock-kneed or are your legs bowed?
   Do your kneecaps face straight ahead?
   Do you lock your knees?
   ++ Your knees should face the same direction as your feet and be slightly relaxed without hyperextending them.
   c. Hips and shoulders: Put your hands on the top of your pelvis so that your thumb faces the rear and your forefinger points down.

* Are hips even or is one higher than the other?

* Does one hip rotate forward of the other?

* Is one shoulder higher than the other?

++ Your hips and shoulders should be even and point straight ahead, like car headlights.

3. **Turn to the side:**

   a. Look at your lower back and tailbone, rest your forefinger in the center of your buttocks, and notice the direction your finger points.

   * If it points straight to the floor, you're in a neutral, balanced position.

   * If it points out behind you, you have an anterior tilt (swayback).

   * If it points under you toward the front, you have a posterior tilt (tucked).

   ++ You should be in a neutral position, tailbone pointing to the floor.

   b. Look at your upper back.

   * Is your upper back rounded and/or rounded at the shoulders?

   * Is your rib cage collapsed or jutting forward?

   ++ Your upper back muscles should be squeezed together so you're straight with shoulder down and relaxed.

   c. Look at your head and neck.

   * Does your chin jut forward?

   * Does your head drop forward?

   * Is your ear in line with your shoulder, hip, and ankle?

   ++ Your head should be in line with your neck; you should be able to draw a line down the side of your body, through your shoulder, hip, and ankle joints.

If your body seems a little "out of whack," make some notes for yourself so you can pay particularly close attention to the exercises in chapters 8-10 that strengthen these muscles. Good posture, like diet and exercise, is just a habit that needs practice.

Priority Training

Health is not a gamble, nor fitness a calculated risk, unless you don't do anything to help yourself. If you choose to eat unhealthily, continue precarious lifestyle habits, and/or avoid exercise, then you're playing Russian roulette with your life.

Changing unwanted habits is difficult. Susan Dey started exercising again when she quit smoking. "I used to exercise in my twenties and stayed fit with diet and exercise; I was my strongest ever for two to three years," Susan said. "When I quit smoking, I missed the "inhale, exhale" breathing so much, I needed to replace it with something. So I started doing aerobics. I could tell myself I was filling my lungs with oxygen instead of cigarette (smoke). But then all the other exercise benefits came with it."

For Susan, the most important thing for her to deal with first was her smoking habit. Adding aerobic exercise to her daily schedule helped her to handle this, which in turn helped with all the other issues in her life, such as stress and getting strong again.

If you did all these little quizzes and activities, you should have a pretty good idea of who you are—physically, that is. Again, the purpose of the self-assessments is to give you a starting point, whether you are starting out for the first time or starting over again, but maybe with a different perspective.

If you have a lot to change, choose your priorities—the items you want to work on first. The rest will come, just like it did for Susan and all my clients. Don't get scared if there's a lot to do; pick what's most important to you and *just start.*

∽

Do it just for today, and if today seems too much, then do it a moment
at a time, a rep at a time, etc., etc., etc.
—Keli Roberts

∽

Real Fitness

Realistic self-assessment, or reflective inventory, means looking at what's there; what's in excess and what's in deficit; then making positive changes. Realistic task setting will be the benefit you will achieve from this process. "Realistic" also needs to be the emphasis of your role model.

Here's an exercise I use with my clients when they begin their program: I'll ask them to find either an old photo of themselves when they felt good about their bodies or a picture of someone they would choose as a realistic and healthy role model. I've found it particularly helpful to have a source of inspiration, something tangible to work toward. Both Cher and Kirstie Alley kept their favorite swimsuit shots of themselves on the fridge; it's an excellent place for yours, too!

One thing I've learned about exercise and health: It's not just a physical experience. No matter how hard I work out in the gym or what positive strides I've made, if I don't feel good about myself when I look in the mirror, I'm still unhappy with me and what I see. I've believed for many years now that my body, mind, and spirit are very much connected, and that it's when I try and disconnect them that I run into problems. Like an equilateral triangle, if I remove one side of the triangle, it will collapse. So I direct my clients and students to take a look at the big picture in finding their own path to balance.

After surviving every conceivable form of eating disorder, and trying so many destructive ways of controlling my weight, I knew I needed to find a more loving—not to mention easier—way of coming to terms with what seemed like an impossible task, which was getting in shape. Without the right method or program or an encouraging instructor, getting in shape *was* an impossible task. But with the right tools, it really isn't impossible; it's completely within your grasp.

∿

STARTING

The two important things I did learn were that you are as powerful and strong as you allow yourself to be, and that the most difficult part of any endeavor is taking the first step, making the first decision.
—*Robyn Davidson, author of* Tracks

∿

The First Step

Here's the good news: You've already taken that first step just by reading this book; you're on the path to change. You've made the decision yourself, and that's truly important when it comes to taking that second step and the third. After years of self-abuse and hiding out, my client Theressa realized that she herself played the biggest part in reversing the same dangerous trap I had fallen into a few years ago.

Theressa said, "I was just yo-yoing around, beating myself up and not getting anywhere. I needed to look clearly at myself in the mirror and say, 'It's time.' I committed when I finally took the time for myself and saw how much I didn't like myself; I wasn't happy. It's all when you're ready; no one can make you ready. I realized I had to *want this*. When I realized I was important, I was ready."

It's been wonderful to watch Theressa's metamorphosis. In about one year, she's lost twenty-four pounds and kept it off. But most importantly, she feels differently about herself. Recently she said to me,

"Before, I hid behind my job and always had the excuse that I had no time. But the reality is that I didn't like who I presented and really didn't want to be out there. Now I'm out there and it feels really good . . . I'm proud because I like who I am now. The biggest improvement is my attitude and how I look at myself. I'm in shape and I look at myself like I'm thin now and I'm not even there yet, so can you imagine when I'm really thin what I'll be like?"

You too can bring about a permanent change. You need to give yourself a pat on the back and just start off real slow. Susan Dey remembers when she first started to work out: "You have to set realistic goals for yourself; otherwise, the first thing we all do is set ourselves up to fail. What worked for me is holding myself to so many minutes of exercise a day. If I choose to go over that, it's great, but tomorrow I don't have to do that many more minutes because then we fall into failure mode. Exercise should be an extension of positive feelings about yourself, not setting yourself up for a negative response."

I couldn't agree with her more.

Notes

Notes

Notes

THREE

Nutrition

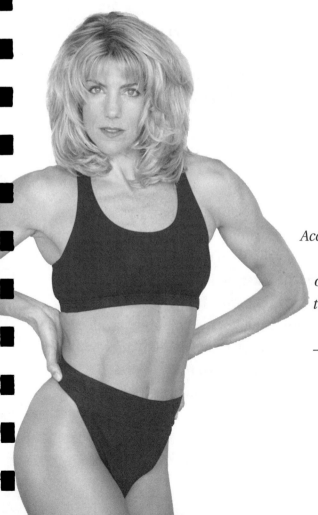

ACTION

*Acceptance is not submission;
it is acknowledgment
of the facts of a situation,
then deciding what you're
going to do about it.*
—Kathleen Casey Theisen

E xercise and diet go hand in hand when it comes to your body as well as your health. Your body will respond to exercise alone, particularly if you've never done it before. But it will respond a whole lot better if you are careful with what you eat. I always consider nutrition a major topic with my clients. You should, too.

Fueling the Fire

There are six basic nutrients for health. Food is fuel composed of all the essential nutrients for maintaining optimal health.

Water

Water is essential to life. It provides a fluid medium for all chemical reactions in the body, the circulation of the blood, and the removal of waste. It is a lubricant and plays a vital role in regulating our body temperature. Our bodies are 70 percent water, and our weight is comprised of 50 to 55 percent water. We need a minimum of eight 8-ounce glasses of water a day. If you live in a warm climate, an environment with central heating, or you fly frequently, you need to add another three or four glasses a day. Working out also will increase your water needs. If you find you don't sweat during your workout, you might be dehydrated or not working hard enough.

So are you thirsty yet? Get ready to drink up.

Learning to drink water didn't come easily to me. For years, people told me that if I drank more water, my skin would clear up. It never made sense to me that drinking water was going to help my skin. Besides, I rarely sweated during my workouts, which I mistakenly thought was something genetic; on top of that, I just didn't like water, period.

Big mistake! How right "they" were! The change in my skin has been nothing short of miraculous. I went from having chronically blemished, "mucky-looking" skin to a glowing, clear complexion, which I predominately attribute to staying well hydrated. Occasionally, I forget to drink enough, and the first symptom I notice is my skin. That's my incentive to drink plenty of water. Oh, by the way, I now also sweat *buckets* when working out.

Cher is so particular about water that she carried cases (and cases and cases) of her preferred brand throughout her entire European tour! We went to thirty-two cities during a two-and-a-half-month period. That's an awful lot of lugging!! But just look at her, a glowing testimony to water!! *Cheers!*

Here are some great tips for becoming more "water conscious":

- When you first get up in the morning, drink sixteen to twenty ounces before you do anything else.

- Invest in a water lug or carrier of some type so you have it with you at all times.

- Always keep a bottle in your car.

- Drink a large glass before every meal.

- Drink during meals. (This will not only increase your water intake; it also will perhaps slow your food intake and help you register how much you're actually eating.)

- Always keep a large bottle on hand whenever you work out, especially during endurance-type activities; take a good gulp every fifteen minutes or so.

- Keep a bottle on your desk at work and take regular "breather sips."

Carbohydrates

Once believed to be the culprit of the dreaded spare tire, we've since found out to the contrary (thank goodness, I just *love* my "carbs"). It's not the pasta, but what we put on the pasta, which maketh the man expand.

Carbohydrates are the best energy source for exercise. With only four calories per gram, they not only fuel your muscles when you are working out, but also "feed" your brain and nervous system. A healthy diet should comprise a minimum of 50-60 percent of your total caloric intake. Foods such as breads, pasta, rice, cereals, grains, and starchy vegetables are ideal. Some form of carbohydrate needs to be included in all three main meals.

Protein

Most of my male clients eat way too much protein, while my females live on carbs and fruit. There's no getting around it; you need protein in your diet, but be careful to get the right amount of it. If you want your muscles to get hard, your mind and concentration clear, your skin and hair healthy, you need to include regular, small amounts of lean protein in your diet.

Excessive amounts of protein do more harm than good, placing strain on the kidneys, which have to excrete excess waste products. Too much protein is also known to increase the loss of calcium in the body. So the key to protein consumption is moderation. Think of it as the supporting act with *vegetables and carbohydrates* in the starring role.

When digested, protein is converted into amino acids, which are used for building and repairing muscles, red blood cells, hair, and other tissues, and for synthesizing hormones. Protein is a source of calories (four calories per gram) and can be used in energy production when there are inadequate carbohydrate stores. This typically happens when calorie intake is too low or during exhaustive exercise. Twelve to 15 percent of your total caloric intake should come from protein-rich foods: chicken, fish, turkey (breast), lean cuts of red meat, and dried beans or legumes.

Fat

Some people think they have a sweet tooth, when in fact they have a "fat tooth." Don't laugh—most of our favorite sweets contain large amounts of fat in conjunction with the sugar. I've never had a particularly sweet tooth. I do, however, have a fat tooth. Just sit me down in front of a bowl of nuts, chips, or buttery popcorn, and watch me go. Actually, I've patiently trained myself not to because I tuned in to how sluggish it makes me feel. My favorite "healthy" sandwich used to be: avocado, cheese, and mayo, with tomato and sprouts—whoops! The whole-wheat bread, sprouts, and tomato got to stay; the rest has since been replaced with turkey, mustard, lettuce, and fat-free mayo. Not only is it delicious, it also contains a much better balance of nutrients.

Fat is a highly concentrated energy source. There are nine calories per gram, so it's easy to end up with a high number of calories in a relatively inconspicuous amount of space! Animal fats (butter, lard, fat in meats) tend to be saturated and are known to cause heart disease, some cancers, high cholesterol, and strokes. Vegetable fats (peanut oil, olive oil, and corn oil) are generally unsaturated and less harmful, although they, too, should still be used in moderation only. They contain the same number of calories per gram. Between 20-25 percent of your total caloric intake should come from fats. *Note:* Not all vegetable fats are unsaturated. A good way to tell is if the fat is hard at room temperature (like coconut), which indicates a saturated fat.

Vitamins

Vitamins are your metabolic controllers, the catalysts which regulate the chemical reactions within the body. In other words, they ensure the smooth running of the engine, without providing any direct source of energy. While vitamins are crucial to the body's processes, they aren't an energy source and they're noncaloric (that's good news!).

Vitamins are classified as either water-soluble or fat-soluble. Water-soluble vitamins B and C are transported by body fluids, with excess excreted in urine. The fat-solubles are A, E, D, and K. Excessive intake of these vitamins can be toxic and harmful, because your body doesn't excrete them like water-soluble vitamins, they're stored in the body's tissues.

Most vitamins are not manufactured within the body; therefore, they need to be obtained through your diet. Well-balanced meals with a variety of foods should be sufficient to meet daily vitamin requirements. While taking megadoses of vitamins is not necessarily better, vitamin deficiency can affect your health and your ability to function at your best. The balance between the various vitamins is delicate and easily upset. Even with the healthiest of habits, it can be difficult to maintain the perfect diet in which we consume the exact balance of nutrients needed. As a safeguard, I sometimes recommend a good multivitamin such as Twin Labs. Remember, though, a supplement is no substitute for a meal; vitamins are more readily absorbed through food sources.

Minerals

My female clients are just the worst when it comes to getting adequate (if any) calcium in their diets. "Dairy products are fattening" is the argument against this nutrient's most valuable source. Big mistake. Whole-milk products are high in fat; calories and cholesterol in this form should be consumed only occasionally and in small amounts. However, low-fat and nonfat counterparts are wonderful alternatives and vital components to a balanced diet. With health concerns such as osteoporosis, women more than ever need to be ambitious with their calcium intake. No supplement is absorbed as well as a food source. If you have difficulty digesting milk products, try Lactaid, which has the lactose removed. Nonfat yogurt is also easy to digest.

Minerals, like vitamins, are not a calorie source and do not provide energy. They are the elements obtained from foods and combine in many ways to create structures of the body. For example, calcium is important for building strong bones and nails; iron increases red blood cell capacity for oxygen transportation. Other important minerals such as magnesium, sodium, potassium, zinc, and phosphorous assist in equally important metabolic processes. Mineral depletion or imbalance as a result of dehydration or an incomplete diet can cause cramps or, if seriously disrupted, an irregular heartbeat.

U.S. RDA Vitamins and Minerals

* The following are the U.S. RDA standards for adults and children over the age of four:

Vitamin A ....5,000 IU
Vitamin C ....60 mg.
Thiamin ....1.5 mg.
Riboflavin ....1.7 mg.
Niacin ....20 mg.
Calcium ....1 g.
Iron ....18 mg.
Vitamin D ....400 IU

This is not a requirement, but rather an estimate of a safe and adequate nutrient intake that maintains good health. Ideally, it is best to try and meet your RDAs on a daily basis; however, if your diet fluctuates, but your weekly average intake meets your allowances, you are unlikely to suffer from any dietary insufficiencies. (Note: If you are a woman over the age of thirty-five or pregnant, these figures may vary.)

Fiber

I like to think of fiber as the "regulator of colon-control intestinal scrub brushes." A high-fiber diet keeps the colon healthy and clean, decreasing the risk of diseases such as diverticulosis and colon cancer. Fiber, which comes from indigestible forms of plant carbohydrates, acts as a bulking agent to add roughage to our diet. You can boost your fiber consumption by eating foods such as fruits and vegetables, whole grains, seeds, nuts, and legumes. Don't link fiber with bloat; although it's possible if you eat an extraordinary amount of fiber and you're not used to it. It's recommended that you include twenty-five to thirty-five grams of fiber daily.

Speaking Of Fiber . . .

Here are a few tips to help you jump on the "Bran Wagon":

- Choose breakfast cereals high in fiber. Fiber One has fourteen grams per cup and contains no sugar; it's also low in sodium and low in calories.

- Fruits—particularly berries, pears, oranges, and kiwis—are rich in fiber. Choose fruits which have edible skins and seeds, because the fiber is generally concentrated in these areas.

- Fresh vegetables which have edible skins and seeds are ideal choices for a fiber-rich diet. Winter squash, broccoli, and spinach are real winners. Whether eaten cooked or raw, the fresh vegetables' fiber content will be approximately the same (although the vitamin content might decrease because of the cooking process in those vegetables high in vitamin C in the raw state).

- Bread and baked goods can be valuable sources when made from the whole-grain flour. Be sure to read the package carefully, as the wrappers can be deceiving. Be wary of bran muffins, as some of these contain up to six hundred calories and more than thirty grams of fat each!

- Legumes and beans, such as lentils and split peas, are not only excellent fiber sources, but also are high in protein and carbohydrates. They make excellent meat substitutes as a way of lowering meat consumption. They are also low in fat. If you find them a little "antisocial," try acclimating your body to them in small, but regular doses. There's also a product called Beano, which contains a digestive enzyme that helps many people (myself included) introduce more fibrous products into their diets without discomfort. The main trick is to introduce them in moderation in order to allow your body an adjustment period. Believe me, it's well worth the patience: not only does fiber keep you regular, but it may protect you from life-threatening diseases.

Our bodies are like engines. What happens if you pour cheap gasoline into your car engine? Doesn't your car just fall apart? We can't keep dumping poison into our bodies from every angle and expect them to keep running properly. Put the right fuel into your body and you'll feel a whole lot better right away.
—*Cher, from* Forever Fit

Food Exchange: The Healthy Eating Alternative

When a client comes to me with a deadline for getting in shape and has to lose a certain number of pounds for a certain role, I find that the food exchange system is the ultimate way to go. Cher used this plan with great success in a very short period of time to get in shape for her videos, as well as for her European tour. When Kirstie Alley needed to quickly drop the thirty-five pounds she had gained for a role she had just finished, this is the plan I put her on, too. It certainly works for me when I have a photo shoot or TV show for which I need to be in my best shape. What I like about it is that it *works fast*!!!

Using food exchanges is the most painless way I've found to lose one to two pounds a week and *not* get hungry. Since it's based on your own personal food preferences, *you* get to choose what you eat. This is all about healthy eating and sticking to a plan. So whatever you eat should be palatable and something you like.

This is not a punishing plan; you don't have to dislike your meals until you're at your desired weight. If your meal was blah and boring, it's because you chose it. It's perfectly acceptable to *enjoy* meals, that's normal and healthy. This isn't an only-at-home, hide-in-the-closet-with-your-measuring-scale diet either. Go out and enjoy a restaurant meal, using the exchanges to guide you. Remember, you're the one making the meal choices, so if you're hungry and not satisfied, change your food combinations for your next meal. If you have trouble understanding portion size, this will definitely teach you how to moderate.

Stop Poisoning Your Body with Food!!!

Too much of anything, no matter what it is—low-fat, low-cal, or otherwise—can make you gain weight. Once ingested, food is either used for energy or stored as fat. If you eat more calories than your body requires, something has to happen to the excess calories your body doesn't use. The result—an expansion in your fat cells.

Food with a high percentage of fat turns to fat more readily. Fat is transported to our cells energetically and efficiently without any caloric expenditure. According to recent research (discussed by Dr. Daniel Cosich during a World Research Forum at the 1994 Idea International Convention in Las Vegas), it appears that fat circulating in the bloodstream stimulates the mechanism which enables our body to more readily store fat. Carbohydrates and proteins are broken down and stored in a different manner. In other words, calorie per calorie, fat is more fattening than carbohydrates or protein. (Another incentive is not to ingest a lot of it in the first place!) A diet with the same number of calories and a larger percentage of fats to carbohydrates causes an increase in fat gain, versus a diet higher in carbs with the same calorie consumption. You'll find the prescribed eating plans further in this chapter very low in fat and very high in fresh vegetables.

Unlike the U.S. Department of Agriculture's food pyramid, you'll find six categories instead of five: the fruit and vegetables are in separate "exchanges." I find this aspect of the plan particularly helpful as a means of becoming "vegetable aware." Clients often come to me eating diets almost exclusively protein, carbs, and fat—no fruit, no veggies. Vegetables are powerhouses of essential nutrients, fiber, and bulk, but without a ton of calories. In fact, you can eat really decent amounts of them without ever needing to be concerned about weight gain. What I've found particularly helpful for fighting feelings of deprivation (often experienced when restricting your intake) is increasing vegetable intake. They provide a pleasant bulk while adding color to your plate, texture to chew, and very few calories ... *this is a very good thing!!!*

Basic Food Group Exchanges

(Adapted by Tobi Levine, MPH, R.D., from the American Dietetic Food Exchanges.)
For each food group, there are "choice equivalents" and the amount of servings you should include in your diet daily for each group. You can *choose* any food in the group, as long as it doesn't exceed the serving recommendation per day. For example, you should include seven servings of starches daily. This doesn't mean you have to eat seven different things, although you can for a well-rounded diet. In one instance, one-half of an English muffin is one serving. If you want a whole English muffin, this counts as two servings. Got it? It's easy to follow. The food exchange system sets up your servings according to portion size and calories per portion. As long as you don't exceed the portion size or number of portions per group, you have free choice.

Starch/Bread/Grain

One serving is approximately 100 calories.

2-3 grams protein: 0 grams fat: 15 grams carb

Key:

c.=cups

cal.=calories

gms.=grams

oz.=ounces

t.=teaspoons

T.=tablespoons

Choose **7** servings from any of the food equivalents below:

1/2 c. starchy vegetables:	1 slice bread
corn, winter squash,	1/2 English muffin
peas, potatoes, beans	1/2 bagel
1/2 c. grain:	1 corn tortilla
pasta, barley,	1/2 flour tortilla
millet, kasha, rice	3/4 c. dry cereal
1/2 c. cooked cereal	4-6 crackers
4 oz. baked potato	3 c. air-popped popcorn
6 oz. veg soup (not creamed)	2 rice cakes

Vegetables

One serving is approximately 25 calories.

2 grams protein: 0 grams fat: 5 grams carb

Choose **4** servings of 1/2 c. cooked or 1 c. raw of the following:

lettuce	tomato	zucchini
mushrooms	onions	turnip
broccoli	pea pods	artichoke
cauliflower	celery	bean sprouts
cabbage	cucumbers	eggplant
asparagus	green/wax beans	beets
water chestnuts	green/red peppers	carrots

| summer squash | collard greens | spinach |

turnip greens

Fruit

One serving is 60-100 calories.

0-1 grams protein: 0 grams fat: 15-25 grams carb

Choose **3-4** servings of any of the following equivalents:

1 fresh, medium fruit:

apple	small pear
orange	persimmon
peach	

1/2 fresh, medium fruit:

| banana | cantaloupe |
| grapefruit | |

3 dates or prunes, 1 oz. raisins

2 figs, apricots, plums, or kiwis; 15 grapes or cherries

1 c. berries

1 1/2 c. melon balls

1/2 c. unsweetened juice, applesauce, or fruit cocktail

Meat/Protein

One serving is 3-4 ounces.

Choose **3** servings from any of the following equivalents:

	gms. protein	gms. fat	gms. carb
lean meat	7	1-3	0
med. fat	7	5	0
high fat	7	8	0

About 150-200 calories:

1/2 whole chicken breast	1 hamburger
1 medium fish fillet	1/2 c. tuna
3/4 c. cottage cheese	

About 75 calories:

1 oz. medium-fat meat	1 oz. low-fat hard cheese
1 egg	

About 50 calories:

1 oz. lean meat, chicken

1 1/2 oz. fish

1 oz. Lite-Line or other nonfat hard cheese

Milk

One serving is 90-120 calories.

Choose **3** servings per day of any of the following equivalents:
1 c. milk:

	gms. protein	gms. fat	gms. carb
skim	9	0	12
low fat	10	5	12
regular	8	8	11

1 c. nonfat milk	1 c. nonfat yogurt
2 oz. nonfat hard cheese	1 c. 1% fat milk
1 c. plain low-fat yogurt	

Fat

One serving is 35-40 calories.

Choose **1** serving per day of any of the following equivalents:
3-5 grams fat

1 t. margarine	1 t. mayonnaise
1 t. oil	1 t. peanut butter
1 t. butter	2 t. diet margarine
2 t. diet mayonnaise	1 T. salad dressing
2 T. diet salad dressing	6-10 nuts
5 large or 10 small olives	1 T. cream cheese
1/8 avocado	

Directions: Copy this sheet so you have one for each day. Fill sheet in, noting the kind of food you ate and the number of exchanges you used.

Daily Meal Plan

_____CALORIES

Number of Exchanges	Kind of Food

BREAKFAST: Time_____
___starch   list 1 _____
___protein   list 2 _____
___vegetables list 3 _____
___fruit   list 4 _____
___milk   list 5 _____
___fat   list 6 _____

MID-MORNING SNACK: Time_____
___   list _____
___   list _____
___   list _____

LUNCH: Time_____
___starch   list 1 _____
___protein   list 2 _____
___vegetables list 3 _____
___fruit   list 4 _____
___milk   list 5 _____
___fat   list 6 _____

Number of Exchanges	Kind of Food

MID-AFTERNOON SNACK: Time_____
___   list _____
___   list _____
___   list _____

DINNER OR SUPPER: Time_____
___starch   list 1 _____
___protein   list 2 _____
___vegetables list 3 _____
___fruit   list 4 _____
___milk   list 5 _____
___fat   list 6 _____

BEDTIME SNACK: Time_____
___   list _____
___   list _____
___   list _____

100-200 Calorie Healthy Energy-Boosting, Low-Fat Snacks:
(Tips from Toby Levine, MPH, R.D.)

Don't forget your snacks!! Healthy eating is more than three solid meals a day. These in-betweeners will really fill the empty gap!

1. Dannon Lite Yogurt (100 cal.) with 2 T. low-fat granola (50 cal): 150 cal.

2. $1^1/_2$ c. frozen grapes (remove from vine, rinse in water, sprinkle with Equal, and freeze): 150 cal.

3. 2 oz. nonfat cheese with 1 oz. (6-10) nonfat or low-fat crackers: 160 cal.

4. 2 oz. nonfat cheese with small apple: 120 cal.

5. 8 oz. nonfat yogurt with 1 c. fresh or frozen berries: 180 cal.

6. 1 c. flaked dry cereal with 4 oz. nonfat milk: 150 cal.

7. $1^1/_2$ oz. pretzels: 150 cal.

8. 4 c. popcorn: between 100-160 cal. (if air or oil-popped)

9. 2 rice cakes with $^1/_2$ c. nonfat cottage cheese and 2 t. low-sugar jam: 170 cal.

10. 2 rice cakes with 2 t. peanut butter and 2 t. honey: 175 cal.

11. Cafe latte with nonfat milk and 2 SnackWell fat-free cookies: 160 cal.

12. Orange-banana smoothie ($1/2$ c. nonfat yogurt, $1/2$ ripe banana, $1/2$ orange, 1-2 t. honey): 175 cal.

13. Strawberry smoothie (made with 8 oz. buttermilk, $1/2$ c. frozen strawberries, and Equal to taste): 175 cal.

14. $1/2$ bagel with 2 T. fat-free cream cheese, onion, and tomato: 125 cal.

15. $1/2$ bagel with tomato and sliced hard-boiled egg with fat-free mayonnaise: 185 cal.

16. $1/2$ turkey sandwich made with 1 slice 100 percent whole-wheat bread, 2 oz. turkey, mustard, and lettuce: 180 cal.

17. $1/2$ cheese sandwich made with 1 slice 100 percent whole-wheat bread, 2 oz. cheese, mustard, and lettuce: 170 cal.

18. 1-2 c. raw vegetables (broccoli, carrots, celery, cauliflower, green pepper) with $1/4$ c. fat-free dip: 150-175 cal.

19. 1 ripe banana with 4 T. nonfat sour cream: 175 cal.

20. $1/2$ sandwich made with 1 slice 100 percent whole-wheat bread, 1 T. peanut butter, 1 t. jam: 190 cal.

21. 2 slices "Vogel" (50 cal. whole-wheat bread) toasted with 2 T. skim milk ricotta cheese and 2 t. low-sugar jam: 150 cal.

22. $1^1/2$ oz. fat-free potato chips: 150 cal.

23. Diet hot chocolate (50 cal.) with 3 fat-free cookies (about 40 cal. each): 170 cal.

24. 6 oz. nonfat frozen yogurt with 2 T. low-fat granola: 170 cal.

25. English muffin with 1 oz. shredded nonfat cheese grilled in oven: 200 cal.

26. 1 oz. trail mix with 4 oz. nonfat Dannon Lite Yogurt: 200 cal.

27. 1 c. fresh or frozen berries with $1/2$ c. nonfat cottage cheese: 150 cal.

28. Tuna & peanut butter snack: 2 oz. tuna with 2 t. peanut butter on caramel rice cake: 190 cal.

29. 8 oz. nonfat milk with 2 fat-free chocolate SnackWell cookies: 190 cal.

Beating the Diet Dilemma

Some people survive really well on a structured eating plan; others don't. This is not a question of strength or weakness. Some of us are more successful learning to slowly modify and replace certain foods in our diets. Others prefer a crash course in nutrition and are mentally prepared to change everything at once. It took me two years to switch from whole milk to skim, which I did via 2 percent, then 1 percent, then skim. It was one of those habits I was not prepared to "plunge" into immediately. Some things are easier than others.

If you're a "wader" when it comes to changing your food habits, patience and unconditional persistence will be the keys to successful modification and replacement. Although results take a little longer, I recommend slow change so as to ensure that your newfound habits naturally become a part of your daily dietary pattern. If you need more immediate changes, you might have to take a deep breath and plunge right into making more serious adjustments in your food choices.

One thing is for sure—the suggestions I've made with the food exchanges are *not* a diet. It's simply a way of learning healthier eating habits with a controlled caloric intake. The great thing about it (apart from being painless and easy) is that it is *permanent* because you learn to understand how to eat according to your needs *and* your preferences. This puts *you* in control—you will learn what and how much you need, and when you need it, and your eating plan will go with you wherever you are, in any situation.

Whatever you do, *don't* skip any meals or snacks. Reducing calories and fat is one thing, eliminating meals is another. Cutting corners by skipping meals isn't going to get you leaner any faster. As a matter of fact, you might hinder yourself from losing weight, because you'll burn calories more slowly. In turn, you're setting yourself up to overeat later from overhunger. When it comes to mealtime, cut down, don't cut out.

Following is the easiest plan you'll ever follow. If you hate dieting; if you feel deprived and end up bingeing on the foods you're doing without; if you are the kind of person who gains weight on a diet; then this is the course of action for you. This is not about overnight changes. Do as much as you're able, then just keep coming back. Keep chipping away.

Baby Steps . . . Big Changes . . . The Gentle Nutrition Makeover

The Intake-Outtake

I will eliminate: automatically eating everything on my plate when eating out.
I will instead: order half portions or share half with a friend.

I will cut back: all fried foods.
I will add: steamed, broiled, baked, and raw foods.

I will cut back: unhealthful snacks.
I will add: healthy substitutes (see "Snack Attack!" for ideas).

I will cut back: high-calorie desserts: cheesecakes, ice cream and sundaes, cakes, etc.
I will add: fresh fruit, $^1/_2$ cup nonfat frozen yogurt, or ice milk.

I will cut back: luncheon meats such as bologna, salami, pastrami, and all mayo-laden chicken and tuna salad sandwiches.
I will add: chicken or turkey breast (skinless),water-packed tuna, or low-fat ham.

I will cut back: high-calorie salad dressings and mayonnaise.
I will add: low- and nonfat substitutes, and take my dressings on the side.

I will cut back: whole milk and other whole dairy products and cheese.
I will add: skim milk or $^1/_2$ percent milk, nonfat cottage cheese, non- or low-fat cheese (read the labels carefully).

I will cut back: butter, margarine, and greasy/oily/fatty foods high in cholesterol.
I will add: small amounts of olive and canola oils (for cooking), and healthier diet margarine varieties (read labels carefully).

I will cut back: large servings of meat and protein.
I will add: small amounts of chicken and fish, lean cuts of red meat (no more than three times per week).

I will cut back: salt (especially adding it at the table), foods containing high quantities of sodium.
I will add: low-sodium substitutes, use more fresh herbs and condiments which are sodium free.

I will cut back: muffins, quick breads, and pastries.
I will add: bagels, low- or nonfat substitutes.

I will cut back: organ meats and sweet breads (they are not only high in fat; they are extremely high in cholesterol).

I will add: more vegetables to my overall intake.

I will cut back: all creamy/butter-based sauces.

I will add: marinara and tomato-based sauces.

I will cut back: nuts (just an ounce can supply anywhere from 13 to 22 grams of fat).

I will add: pretzels or baked corn chips.

I will cut back: sugar, sweets, and candies (vending machines and "free" samples count!).

I will add: sugarless substitutes.

I will eliminate: frying foods in butter or lard.

I will instead: use a nonstick skillet with a Pam-type spray and a low-sodium fish or chicken stock.

I will eliminate: eating the skin on chicken and the fat on red meat.

I will instead: cut it off before eating it or, if the temptation is too great, before cooking it.

I will eliminate: rich creamy sauces such as hollandaise, bernaise, beurre blanc, or gravy.

I will instead: choose thin, stock-based sauces or tomato (red) sauces.

I will eliminate: refined, processed foods typically low in fiber.

I will instead: include more fiber in my diet by choosing foods which are naturally fibrous.

The Bottom Line on Metabolism

The big question any time you're trying to change your eating habits is: *How much is enough?* One way to find out how much food you really need is to calculate your basal metabolic rate (BMR). Your BMR is the amount of calories you need at rest; it's the amount of calories your body requires to function metabolically. When you're more active in your daily life or you exercise, your body needs more calories to maintain its base level. When you're more sedentary, you don't use as many calories. If you're more muscular, you have a higher BMR and you more efficiently burn calories. To maintain your current weight, you need to eat as many calories as your body requires, depending upon your daily activity. To lose weight, you need to be in the negative, you need to eat less than your BMR requirement.

Now, when it comes to food, here's the bottom line: In order to *gain* one pound of fat, you have to eat thirty-five hundred calories in *excess* of your base needs. That's where the term "creeping fat" came from; over a period of time, those excess calories just creep up on you—on your hips, on your thighs, and wherever else fat lies. If you went out to dinner and weighed yourself the next morning and your scale weight was one pound heavier, you would have to have eaten thirty-five hundred extra calories the day before (that's equal to either six and a half Big Macs, six banana splits, 117 slices of bacon, twenty-six donuts or forty-six slices of bread). Guess what? You didn't get "fatter" overnight just because you went out to dinner and splurged a little; extra water weight is the more common culprit. But if splurging continues on a daily basis, the calories add up over a period of time.

The same theory works in reverse, if you want to *lose* one pound you have to reduce the number of calories in your diet by thirty-five hundred calories. You can do this by diet alone—reducing your intake by five hundred calories per day so that you'll lose one pound in one week. *Or* you can reduce your calories with a combination of exercise and diet. Reducing your diet by 250 calories a day is pretty easy, once you start looking for where those hidden calories are. Making healthier eating choices and using the food exchange plan will help you. Then, by adding thirty minutes to an hour of daily exercise or activity, by the end of one week, you should be in a thirty-five-hundred-calorie deficit. Pretty painless, isn't it? However, don't justify balancing your three-hundred-calorie piece of cake with a three-hundred-calorie Stairclimber workout the same day; the skinny on calories is that in the end, it's the total that counts. The checks and balance is with *total* input-output, not on an item-to-item basis.

To figure your BMR use the following chart. It involves a little bit of calculating and math, but it will help you get perspective on how many calories your body *really* needs to survive. You might be surprised. If you need to lose weight, once you know you're BMR, you can reduce the number of calories per day through a daily reduction in calories and by adding exercise. If you have an active lifestyle, you'll be surprised how efficient your body really is. Don't forget, it's "total calories in equals total calories out" for maintenance; "total calories out *minus* total calories in" for weight loss.

A Simplified Method For Rough Estimation of Daily Energy Needs

Here is a simple four-step method of making a rough estimate of daily energy needs in kilocalories (kcal: usually called calories).

First Step: (Estimate basal metabolic energy needs [BMR])

1. Change pounds to kilograms:
    weight in pounds/2.2 = weight in kilograms
    Example: A 150-pound woman
    150/2.2 = 68 kg.

2. Multiply kg weight times BMR factor:
    1.0 kcal/kg/hr. for males
    0.9 kcal/kg/hr. for females
    Example: 68 x 0.9 = 61 kcal per hour

3. Multiply the kcals used in one hour by 24 (hours in a day)
    Example: 61 x 24 = 1,464 kcal/day BMR

Second Step: (Estimate physical activity energy needs)

4. Determine % of BMR depending on lifestyle in terms of muscular activity
    Example: Our 150-pound woman is a sedentary typist:
    1,464 kcal/day x .20 = 293 cal per day for physical activity

    a   Sedentary person (mostly sitting) add 20% of BMR
    b   Light activity (2-3 days of exercise) add 30% of BMR
    c   Moderate activity (3-5 days of exercise) add 40% of BMR
    d   Heavy work (5-6 days of exercise, athlete) add 50% of BMR

5. Add BMR kcal and activity kcal
   Example: 1,464 + 293 = 1,757

Third Step: (Estimate energy need for specific dynamic effect of food [SDE]—the energy spent on digestion and metabolism of food)

6. Find 10% of total kcals per day in step 5
   Example: 1,757 x 10% = 176 kcal

Fourth Step: (Determine full day's estimated energy needs)

7. Add kcals for BMR, physical activity, and SDE
   Example: BMR = 1,464
   Activity = 293
   SDE = 176
   24 hr. total = 1933 kcal

∾

It's not WHAT you're eating, it's what's eating YOU.
—Keli Roberts

∾

Dealing with Deprivation

One of the main reasons diets don't work is because of the deprivation syndrome. You know it: You're at the dinner table, and everyone else is sitting there having the food you want but "can't" have because you're on a diet. So maybe you resist that day, but the next day at the office, everyone is eating chocolate chip cookies, and they're your favorite. You're already hurting from missing your favorite dessert last night; you're having a hard day at the office; your boss just yelled at you; you had your diet lunch; and it's 2:00 P.M. and *you're hungry*!

What happens all too often, which ends up sabotaging us, is the Deprivation Binge: You have one cookie and decide you've blown it, so you end up eating the whole box . . . eeeekk!!! So now you have to deprive yourself even more, and you try even harder to perfectly follow your diet, meanwhile punishing yourself for your cookie plunder.

Instead, try this: On the evening you want to be included in the family celebration with the special treats, try having the smallest portion, or sharing your portion with someone. Or try replacing it with a healthy substitute.

Another way in which we can easily end up feeling deprived is when we're not getting our emotional needs met and then attempt to replace what's missing with food. How often do you find yourself at the fridge when actually all you're feeling is lonely? Or you find yourself facedown in greasy, salty popcorn when you're angry with someone you need to speak to concerning a touchy situation. The chocolate Haagen Daz is hardly a love replacement! Yet in some ways, it seems easier to turn to the ice cream. For starters, the ice cream won't reject you or hurt your feelings like the handsome guy or pretty girl you've been wishing would even notice you. The "food solution" feels safer.

My client Hank, who is in great shape, told me some sound advice from a psychiatrist she knew: "Don't ever try to fill that void with food, but rather accept the void for what it is . . . a void—that part that was missing from your life. Own it and come to understand it, rather than filling it with food or whatever obsession; see it as a void so you can develop alternative things to do, to compensate for that loss, whatever it is."

Working too hard and taking no time out for yourself can leave you feeling resentful and angry at the world for not fulfilling your needs. How easy is it to come home from work feeling tired and unappreciated, then flop on the couch only to reward yourself with potato chips (you're hungry now and too tired to cook anything, especially after a particularly hard day)? After consuming the entire package, you feel really guilty, having blown your healthy eating resolution, so then you decide that the potato chips are going to be your dinner. Unfortunately, a couple of hours later, you find yourself still on the couch and hungry again, so you figure that you didn't really have any dinner, so dessert won't hurt, so you again find yourself facedown in the Haagen Daz.

Vicious cycle.

What I've found that has worked well for my clients is to learn to be more assertive at the office, make sure work is delegated correctly, and get their own needs met in terms of hours. Sticking up for ourselves not only helps our working situation, but also our eating habits. This type of prioritizing might also help you. If you identify with this scenario, an honest look at what is going on could definitely break this destructive cycle.

Seeking Support

If my clients' goals are weight related, the issues of food and eating habits both need to be addressed. We are all different, so when designing a nutrition program, I first assess the person's eating history to make sure he or she doesn't have more serious concerns involving food. Anorexia, bulimia, or compulsive overeating are surprisingly common among potential clients who are looking for a lifestyle change.

Long-standing food problems might be damaging to your health. In those cases, I suggest seeking professional help in conjunction with exercise. There's lots of help available, ranging from therapy to twelve-step programs. I know for myself, getting the emotional support I needed was every bit as important as getting in shape. It was a bit of a "catch-22"—without the emotional help, I was unable to stick with my exercise program. But working out made the emotional hurdles so much easier to handle.

Behavioral Changes for Permanent Weight Loss

The following activities and behavioral changes have worked for me as well as my clients. They involve food, eating, cooking, and preparation. Take what you like and leave the rest. Be honest; remember, the only one you cheat is yourself.

Do your best with initiating the changes. Some you'll find easier than others. Habits are not easy to change. Some will be so second nature you're probably not even aware you're doing them. Just like "Baby Steps, Big Changes . . . " all you need is the willingness to want to change.

This is not a diet . . . this is about permanent changes in your habits and attitudes toward food and eating.

I will eliminate: eating large portions.
I will instead: listen to my body and feel physically how much is adequate.

I will eliminate: eating quickly and gulping my meals.
I will instead: chew slowly, consciously, putting my fork down between each bite, taking at least twenty minutes to complete the meal.

I will eliminate: eating in the car, at the desk, in front of the TV, or in any other distracting situation.

I will instead: eat meals at locations selected specifically for that purpose (restaurants, cafeterias, dining rooms, etc.).

I will eliminate: eating out of pots and pans, fast-food carry-out containers, serving dishes.

I will instead: eat on smaller, attractive plates with my food appetizingly arranged.

I will eliminate: second helpings.

I will instead: serve the food in the kitchen, not at the table where I'm more tempted to pick or take seconds or even thirds (gulp!).

I will eliminate: eating large amounts of *seemingly* low-calorie foods, such as movie popcorn.

I will instead: be honest with myself about what's really going in my mouth and choose a more appropriate choice and amount. Who are you kidding?

I will eliminate: grocery shopping while hungry. It's easier to fall prey to inappropriate choices and old habits with low blood sugar.

I will instead: shop from a list, buying things from my new healthy choice food plan. It's easier to say "no" in the supermarket than in your fridge.

I will eliminate: hanging out at the buffet table at parties picking, picking, picking . . . endless grazing is best for cows!

I will instead: eat sitting down; then, when finished, get involved in conversations, dancing, or whatever is going on around me which doesn't involve eating.

I will eliminate: "cleaning my plate" at meals, especially in restaurants where the portions are beyond polite!

I will instead: leave the excess. If you know you can't do this, ask for the doggy bag first. I find this particularly helpful with the servings of protein that have a tendency to be way more than what's needed.

I will eliminate: eating more now because I'm scared I'll get really hungry later.

I will instead: have faith that I'll make it to my next meal or snack (in approximately three to four hours). At worst I can add an extra piece of fruit or a caffeine-free diet soda.

I will eliminate: eating any type of food for the sake of social pressure, real or imagined. (Often we place unrealistic pressures on ourselves when, in fact, all we need to do is assert ourselves, ask for what we need, and not worry about what people think. Let 'em . . . It's *your* body . . . not theirs!!!)

Notes

Notes

Notes

Notes

FOUR

Getting Started

Or Restarted

PERSISTENCE
*Continuous effort, not
strength or intelligence, is the
key to unlocking our
potential.*
—Liane Cordes

N ow begins the real fun; planning your personal fitness program. But where do you begin, right? Start with what you enjoy, meaning those activities that give you pleasure, let you relax, or allow you to explore. Variety is important in your life. Ask Cher. She has a versaclimber, treadmill, recumbent bike, rower, and stair-climber in her at-home gym, as well as steps, weight equipment, and practically every other kind of available fitness toy (not to mention her tennis court and pool). Most of us aren't quite so lucky!!

Part of the reason that Cher and I connected so well as client and trainer has to do with the variety I created in her workouts. Although she owned all the necessary equipment and more, she relied on me to constantly challenge and change her routines—depending on her moods, energy, and time constraints. As someone dedicated to life-long fitness, Cher fully understands the mental as well as the physical benefits of a varied program.

Even then, Cher is only human. Like all the rest of us, she sometimes would fall into the humdrum trap. When she discovered something new that she really liked, she would focus in on only that one thing at the expense of variety. Knowing that, I would do all that I could think of to make sure she got right back to doing different things so that she wouldn't burn out on that one new interest. There is a lesson here: Instead of getting stuck on some new exercise or training device, we need to learn to discipline ourselves a little and make sure there's balance.

I *love* outdoor activities, so to supplement my gym workouts, I would ride my bike to the pool, swim my laps, dry off, and then run. Although I adore running, I made it a point to vary my runs to keep from getting bored. On some days, I'd run the stairs nearby or I'd run to the Sydney opera house—my favorite route of all. Other times, I'd change my pace and do a fast walk around the duck pond of the botanical gardens, where I could hear the birds and see the flowers. It was so beautiful and peaceful there, I didn't even realize I was exercising. For a real change of scenery, I'd go to the beach, swim in the surf, and run on the sand. Get the picture? None of this cost anything, either.

Fitness Improv

Exercise shouldn't be a drudgery. It might feel that way when you're first starting, because you're not used to *thinking* about including it. After awhile, however, exercise will become part of your daily life, and you won't *need to think* about putting it on your "to do" list anymore. Adding exercise will make everything else in life seem easier in the process. Exercising is the best stress reliever.

My client Anita, sixty-four, oversees a very successful, time-demanding business with a partner and an eleven-person staff. But she manages to budget enough time to take walks, participate in step classes, and train with weights.

She told me, "The business is always stressful anyway, but with my partner away on vacation, I have to work twelve hours a day and handle the whole office by myself. If I didn't work out with you three days a week, I don't know how I'd handle the stress."

Part of fitting in fitness is being flexible with yourself, attending to your needs, listening to your body, and tuning in to your mind. Susan Dey is an early bird and prefers morning workouts. With her hectic schedule, she sometimes has to make the choice of working out at a different time or skipping it altogether.

"I'm not used to working out at four in the afternoon," Susan said, "but if I can make myself do it, I feel so energized—the only inspiration I know is to do it, knowing the effect it has on you."

I've developed the activity assessment questionnaire to help you outline your workout priorities and how much time you're willing to commit to it. Like the self-assessments in chapter 2, there's no right or wrong here; just give a little thought to what's best for you.

Activity Assessment Questionnaire

Answer the following questions to help you develop your personal fitness program:

1. What physical activities do you like to do; i.e., running, biking, rowing, boxing? _____

2. How much time can you commit each week to exercise; i.e., one hour, four times a week? _____

3. Do you prefer a particular time of day for your workout; i.e., morning or late afternoon? _____

4. Would you rather work out (1) alone, (2) with a partner, or (3) with a group? _____

5. Would you rather exercise (1) indoors or outdoors, (2) in a gym or at home, or (3) vary your workout place? _____

6. What equipment and facilities are available to you?
    (1) full-service gym _____
    (2) free weights only _____
    (3) cardio equipment _____
    (4) none_____
    (5) other _____

7. Does weather affect your workout; i.e. heat, cold, rain? _____
   If yes, what changes do you make? _____
   _____

8. What are your top fitness goals (from chapter 1)
   1. _____
   2. _____
   3. _____
   4. _____

9. What recreational or sport activities do you enjoy that can include your significant other, best friend, children, or other family members? _____

10. What are some new activities that you'd like to try but you haven't?
    _____

If your daily schedule is already action packed, even without an exercise regimen, this assessment will help you see *where* and *how* you can fit it all in. At first you might have to actually block off time in your appointment book. No excuses. Give yourself the permission to take the time.

Before you make any final decisions, take the self-evaluation quiz on page 97. Use the Life Circle on page 100 to help you balance this whole process—work, daily responsibilities, and play—so that you can make healthy lifestyle choices that support, not defeat you. Once you get started, you'll stay started . . . and continue.

❧

BALANCE

*It is basically: how to remain whole in the midst of the distractions of
life; how to remain balanced, no matter what centrifugal forces tend
to pull one off center; how to remain strong, no matter what shocks
come in the periphery and tend to crack the hub of the wheel.*
—*Anne Morrow Lindbergh*

❧

Healthy Choices:
Personalizing Your Fitness Plan

Your answers to the following self-evaluation quiz will guide you in
making some healthy, balanced choices. Everyone needs downtime,
playtime, social time, and solitary time, along with everyday work and
responsibilities. Fitness isn't just physical—it's fitness of the mind as
well. Sometimes a fifteen-minute power nap will do more to energize
you than the thirty-minute Stairmaster workout you struggled through
because you didn't listen to your needs.

This quiz, together with the activity assessment, will help you recognize those things you like to do as well as what's missing. You'll notice
that this circle is perfectly round, with ten equal sections. Based on
your own needs, start anywhere in the circle and determine how big
you need each section. Identify in the Life Circle each of these specific
areas from the following questions and begin to "round out" your life.
Write your comments and answers in the space provided below each
set of questions:

Self-Evaluation Quiz

1. **Why do you want to get fit?**

   Does exercise make you feel great today or are you "waiting" until you look perfect—whenever that is—to enjoy it? Are you in the here and now and experiencing every step of the way, or is there a time when you're hoping exercise will feel better?

   _____
   _____
   _____
   _____
   _____

   Choose activities that will help you enjoy the present ... If you're an environmentalist, do your program out-of-doors. If you're having trouble focusing, try meditation or an activity that's active but also more mental, like yoga.

2. **How much stress do you have in your life right now?**

   Does your job, family, illness, or marital problems cause added worry and distress to your already harried life?

   _____
   _____
   _____
   _____
   _____

   Choose exercises that will let your mind concentrate on what your body is doing, like ballet or martial arts. If you're too stressed to be still, try exercises that are stress stiflers such as boxing or weight training—you still get to concentrate on you, but the activity level is high. If you need to calm your mind, try exercise that will put you into a meditative state: running, stretching. Be flexible and do what feels good at the moment, even if it changes what you had planned.

3. **In what kind of surroundings do you spend most of your day?**
   Are you indoors in a large office with a lot of hustle or do you work in solitude at home? Do you work in a high-tech room without a view or do you have the freedom to be outdoors? Would you describe your daily environment as cluttered or clean?

   _____

   _____

   _____

   _____

   _____

   If you spend most of your time indoors, whether in a large office or at home, choose fresh-air activities such as jogging, mountain biking, roller blading, or outdoor sports—something that will clear your mind. If the computer is your mate most of the day, steer away from high-tech equipment; you get enough of this every day.

4. **Do you spend most of your day talking on the phone, dealing with other people or kids, or are you free from most constant daily interaction?**

   _____

   _____

   _____

   _____

   _____

   If your job is spent primarily with people or constant office noise, give yourself some solitary time with activities that focus on you for a change such as yoga, jogging, tai chi, hiking, gardening, swimming, or meditation. On the other hand, if you spend your days working alone, social stimulus is a must: try team sports, tennis, classes at the gym, dance classes.

5. **Are you a workaholic, a regimented exerciser, or stuck in an exercise rut?**

   Do you spend your day in a structured setting with set breaks, set mealtimes, set exercise schedules; in other words, do you live your life by the clock?

   _____

   _____

   _____

   _____

   _____

   If you're in the same-old, same-old mold, you need some variety and relaxation in your life! Try a different sport or an activity you've been dying to do for a long time but never got around to it. Or the key may be adding some recreation and cultural stimulation. Take a drive with a friend without a map or set plans where you'll go or what time you're expected to be there; go to the movies, visit an art gallery . . . you need playtime.

LIfe Circle

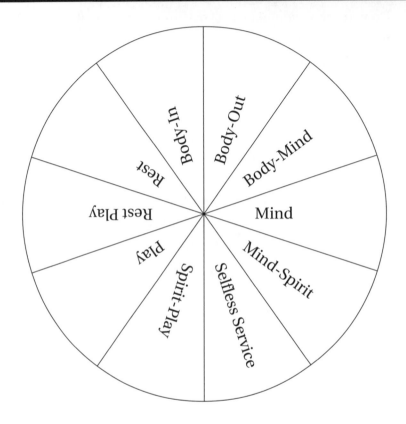

Body-In: Therapeutics: massage, chiropractic and physical therapies, healthy balanced nutrition, water, spa services, and treats.

Body-Out: Cardiovascular exercise: aerobics, step, biking, cross-country skiing, stairclimbing, in-line skating, running, rope jumping. Resistance: weight training, muscle conditioning. Flexibility: stretch classes, yoga.

Body-Mind: Self-defense, competitive sports, activities requiring focus: yoga, martial arts, dance, rock climbing, pilates, stretching.

Mind: Education: seminars, courses in health education, cooking, nutrition and diet, nonfiction books.

Mind-Spirit: Visualization, journaling, psychotherapy, support groups, twelve-step programs.

Selfless Service: Helping others in need, donating time and effort, unconditional giving and care, religious worship, meditation, music.

Spirit-Play: Artistic hobbies: painting, beading, sewing, etc. Gardening: watering, pruning, weeding. Improvisation games, home puttering, family time, solitary time, hiking, and easy outdoor biking.

Play: Theme parks, building sand castles, noncompetitive sports: in-line skating, jog-walks, Frisbee, walking the dog.

Rest-Play: Cultural: art galleries, museums, concerts, ballet, movies. Slow strolls, picnics, social gathering, kite flying, fishing, visiting the zoo.

Rest: Sleep, spas and steams, gentle massage, nonactive time-out, naps and power naps, long baths and showers.

Gearing Up

Having the proper footwear, clothing, and equipment can definitely make exercising a pleasant if not more enhancing experience. Nothing is worse than trying to enjoy a workout, play a sport, or even go for a walk if you're uncomfortable. Here are some tips:

Clothing

Wear comfortable clothing that gives you freedom to move. If you're exercising outdoors, wear something that's well ventilated and light in color. If you're hiking or mountain biking, you might want to wear something long-sleeved to protect you from getting scratched.

Layering your clothing is the best way to acclimate to all weather conditions, particularly in winter. Natural fibers such as cotton and silk are the most breathable when you sweat so that perspiration doesn't cling to your body. When I run outdoors, I find layering my clothes really gives me the freedom to adapt to the wind and cold, without overbundling. Start with a thin layer, like a cotton tank or jog bra closest to your skin. Layer on top of that something like a T-shirt or a light sweatshirt, then a light jacket that you can tie around your waist when it gets hot.

Also, silk long underwear is absolutely fantastic because it's so light and soft against your skin, and any outer gear fits well over it. If it's really cold, wear a lightweight but warm ski turtleneck shirt to keep your neck warm. Wear something over your mouth to humidify the air. One more thing, if it's cold, don't forget to cover your head and hands; you can lose a lot of body heat by staying uncovered and ungloved.

Whatever you choose to wear, stay away from rubberized or plastic clothing. Fat doesn't melt away with sweat. Overheating your body by wearing unventilated clothing can cause dehydration, a major problem during cardiovascular exercise. Dehydration can lead to death. Stick to cotton, because it won't stick to you.

In the summer, definitely go lightweight; you want to avoid getting overheated. Layering is great for summer as well, although you probably will wear fewer layers. Remember, *comfortable* and *protected* are the keys. Active wear with modern fabrics and styles are readily available today, and designed specifically for sport wear and tear.

Shoes

No two feet are alike, not even yours. Choosing the correct shoes is an individual thing and not every shoe is best for every activity. If you're exercising three to five hours a week and involved in a variety of activities, a pair of supportive cross-training shoes would probably suit you. If you're running more than four miles a week, however, invest in a good pair of running shoes; don't run in your cross-trainers. Cross-trainers have a lot of features designed specifically for multipurpose use and might not be the best if you're specializing in any one area of fitness. The same would be true if you're taking a lot of aerobic or step classes, or if you play a racquet sport. Each of these activities requires a certain kind of support and stabilization.

Get some expert advice from a reliable shoe store that specializes in sport shoes. They can measure your foot, check your gait, and test for the kind of support you personally need for the sport that you want to play. Most importantly, buy according to fit, *not* according to brand. Your feet will know the difference.

Shoe design is a high-technology business. For example, running shoes are designed for different foot shapes as well as for different foot strikes, running surfaces, and total miles to be ran. The same is true of hiking boots, aerobic shoes, or walking shoes. If you're doing high-impact aerobics, buy shoes specifically designed for high impact; not only will you protect your feet, but your knees and spine as well. Regardless of your shoe type, here are some basic buying guidelines:

1. Measure both feet; choose the size that fits your larger foot.

2. You should have room to wiggle your toes with about a half-inch

of space at the tip.

3. Shoes should be comfortable when you try them on, not stiff.

4. Make sure you have plenty of support across your instep and the arch support is in the right place for your foot.

5. Try on your shoes with the socks you plan on wearing.

6. Notice the places that you wear down on your regular shoes; for example, this could be on the inside of the heel or the outside. This shows how you distribute your weight when you walk.

7. Make sure you tell the shoe technician what kinds of activities you'll be doing so he can recommend the best shoe for you.

Does this mean you need to have ten pairs of shoes if you're going to do ten different activities? No, but you should have specific shoes for the activities that you do a lot, say, at least three to four hours a week. One final word on shoes: For longer wear, don't wear your indoor workout shoes outside. It's a bother to change them, but they'll last a lot longer if you do.

Sweat Essentials: Water

Drink plenty of water. Then drink more. Need I say more? The trick with outdoor training is that you have to carry water with you if you aren't going to be around a water source. You really need to be conscious about it; it's easy to forget if you're used to training indoors where a water fountain or the sink is right there. There are some great strap-on water carriers nowadays that are really convenient and comfortable. Get one or two. Regardless of where you train, make sure that you're drinking at least three ounces of cool water for every twenty minutes of exercise. I say cool water, because it absorbs more readily without causing stomachaches.

Sweet Inspirations: Walkmans

I must confess, even in the beautiful and great outdoors, I find it hard to be motivated without my music, so I always have a Walkman carrier with me. Same thing for when I exercise. I roller blade with my music, ride the bike, and even weight train with it. It's my starter button; somehow I can't get going without it. Lots of people are like that, too.

Listening to music when I exercise really gives me the space, the solitary time for me, because I spend so much of my day with other people doing their workouts. My music makes it something special for me. A word of caution, however: If you're listening to music in a high-traffic area, whether you're skating or running or just walking, *be careful.* Don't blast your music so loud that you can't hear what's going on in your surroundings; it's dangerous. A good rule of thumb is to set your volume level low enough so that you can still hear normal conversation thirty feet away. Otherwise, you can easily be hit or walk out in front of a car listening to your favorite song.

I was hit by a car once while riding my bike and tuning in to my Walkman. I was listening to Andreas Vollenweider, and I was in a deep meditative state. I rode right into the side of a car. I was so deeply involved in my music, I wasn't "present." Needless to say, my spiritual awakening received a rude awakening. When you get into that "celestial," alpha state, it's very easy to become unaware of cars, dogs, fences . . . whatever. Stay mentally present when you're training outdoors, whether you're listening to music or not.

Supplemental Gadgets: Heart-Rate Monitors

Heart-rate monitors are a really useful tool, even if you're well trained. A good one will keep you on track so you'll know when to speed up or slow down. They work particularly well if you have a hard time getting your heart rate up into your training heart-rate range, or if you're the kind of person that works out too hard. You know, people often think they have to be really breathless to be making gains. The theory, "If you can't speak a sentence, you're probably working too hard," is a misconception.

On the other hand, if you can speak more than a paragraph, you need to pick up your pace. A monitor will precisely help you maintain the correct intensity.

If you're pregnant, it's imperative to train with a heart-rate monitor because your *perceived* exertion is not as accurate when you're pregnant. One of my clients, Marjorie, trained with me all the way through her pregnancy. She'd had fairly easy first and second trimesters, and didn't have problems training and keeping her heart rate within normal ranges for what she was doing.

One day, when Marjorie was just over six months pregnant, I noticed during our session that her heart rate was elevating without lowering again—even during her rest periods—although she *felt* fine. Every time we trained after that, her heart responded by elevating the same way for the rest of her pregnancy. The interesting thing to me was that she didn't notice any difference in how she felt, even though her heart rate was elevated. This was because she was so accustomed to the exercise.

With weight training in particular, whether you're pregnant or not, your heart rate can elevate surprisingly high without any obvious signs that you're overtraining. What's the bottom line? It's easy to be deceived by intensity, even if you're well trained. Cher's sister was working out regularly on a Stairmaster, trying to lose weight without any results. We were surprised to find out how overly high her heart rate was once she started wearing a monitor. Once she lowered her intensity a little and began working in her training range, she immediately began to lose weight. Using a heart-rate monitor is a valuable tool to help you understand the inner workings of your cardiovascular system more clearly, keeping you at the correct workout level.

Weight-Training Gloves

Gloves are really comfortable, particularly if you're doing pulling movements. You don't need gloves to weight train, but they can help you grip a bar or weight more securely. A lot of my women clients like to wear a glove that protects their hands from calluses. If calluses and rough spots are a concern for you, then invest in a good pair of gloves. What I like even better are neoprene grips; they're small three-by-three-inch squares of neoprene. I find grips are less confining than gloves. I can use them for the exercises I want, then easily put them aside.

Weight-Training Belts

Whether you should or shouldn't use a weight belt is one of those gray-area questions; other trainers might have a different opinion. Using a belt to stabilize your spine really takes the place of your own muscles doing the work. I notice that when people *do* use a weight belt, they wear it much too often and for too many exercises. They are far too reliant on it. Doing exercises without a belt "teaches" your abdominals and other torso muscles how to contract to stabilize themselves. So when you go out into your daily life, these muscles are well conditioned with a degree of strength that's specific to your needs.

No client of mine wears a weight belt, although I have some clients with bad backs. There's a good reason for this. If you have a bad back and you're doing an exercise that requires you to wear a belt, there's probably a better position for you to be exercising in that doesn't place as much stress on your back.

I recently started working with a male client who had a bad back and was "addicted" to his weight belt when he exercised. He believed the belt would enable him to lift more weight; but even with it, his form was terrible, his muscles weren't getting any stronger, and his back *still hurt*. Once I weaned him from using his weight belt—by having him practice stricter lifting form in more stabilized positions (so his muscles could actually work harder)—he threw away his belt. He realized he had been cheating for years and not getting any benefit from it. More importantly, his back pain disappeared. Using a weight belt might *seem* like a helpful thing to do, but my advice is to use your muscles instead.

Sundries: Band-Aids

If you're going out hiking, roller blading, or somewhere far from home, always carry a couple of Band-Aids with you in your pocket or your pack. There's nothing like an untimely blister to leave you hobbling and spoil your workout. It's no fun, believe me. Don't leave home without them.

Sun Protection: Glasses, Hats, and Sunscreen

I've always loved the sun. I love being outdoors. I love the beach. I'm a true-blue Aussie! But I'm "sun smart." Don't forget to protect yourself. Use sunscreen liberally; make sure you don't miss your ears and the back of your neck! Wear a cap or hat with a visor to protect your head and face, particularly if you're walking or biking. If you're wearing sunglasses, make sure that they're plastic and not real glass, in case you slip and fall.

Sweatbands and Towels

Some women hate sweating, even the thought of sweating; perhaps its something to do with the "men sweat, women glow" myth. I've seen women drying their leotard off in the locker room in the middle of their workout to disguise it. Let's face it, unsightly sweat lines aren't the signs of a marked woman, but the indication of good health and fitness. Cher, for example, sweats buckets; I've never seen anything like it. She doesn't wear a sweatband when she exercises—she wears a diaper around her head so she can see during her session. To me, Cher is the epitome of femininity!

   If you've never really sweated much before, get ready for a change. That doesn't mean you'll sweat buckets, too, although your body might surprise you. Sweating is your body's cooling system; think of it as your own natural air conditioner, which dissipates body heat. Once your fitness improves and you become more energy efficient, your sweating mechanism might increase to cool you down. This is healthy and normal.

To keep sweat from getting too soppy and to keep you more comfortable, have a towel handy. During weight work, it's good gym etiquette to keep the weight benches dry (I sweat a ton, so I always use a towel). Proper use of a towel is more sanitary and your hands won't lose their grip during training. If you're a "head sweater," use a headband—a bandanna will do—to keep sweat out of your eyes. Makeup and hair products can really sting your eyes; a headband helps you clear the view.

∾

The FITT Formula

When I first started exercising, I had no idea there was a method to figuring out how much I was supposed to do, how hard I was supposed to work out, or how often I could do it. I'm the kind of person that once I make up my mind to do something, I jump in with both feet. No standing on the edge for me. Sound familiar?

Four general principles apply to any cardiovascular training program, and together they form the acronym FITT. This stands for **F**requency, **I**ntensity, **T**ime, and **T**ype. We use the FITT principle for all forms of training; however, each of these variables are applied specifically, depending on what kind of activities you're doing—aerobic, resistance, or flexibility training. Right now, we're going to talk specifically about aerobic training. All four of these principles provide what is called *overload*—supplying stimulus for cardiovascular improvements. By increasing any one of these variables within your program (after your starting point becomes comfortable), you can increase your overload, thus forcing your heart and lungs to work a little harder.

Frequency means how many times a week you exercise. For best aerobic training results, exercise at least three to five times a week. If you're just starting out, take a day off in between, for recovery. Everybody, no matter how fit, needs to take at least one day a week off for rest. Rest can mean sleep. You can be a couch potato if you want, but you can go back to the Life Circle on page 100 and choose some light activity from mind-body, recreation, or rest. Sometimes puttering around the house is my favorite way of "chilling out." Puttering is therapy for me.

Intensity means how hard you're working. Your intensity should be at 55 to 85 percent of your estimated maximum heart rate within five minutes after you begin. You should be able to maintain approximately the same intensity throughout your whole program. You learned how to monitor your heart rate in chapter 2 (page 34). You can also use a heart-rate monitor to be really sure. As your body becomes more aware of how exercise feels, you'll be able to tune into your body's responses and use them as a guide for how hard you're working. This is called "perceived exertion." How hard you're working is really important because it affects your metabolism, energy levels, and ability to burn calories. Stay within your range. You'll feel much better if you do.

Time means how long your aerobic session should be. To maximize aerobic benefit, exercise for at least twenty, and up to sixty continuous minutes. Here's the catch: If you work out *too hard*, you might not be able to work out for very long, because it's too intense. For example, if you're accustomed to working out for twenty minutes, and you want to increase your duration to twenty-five minutes, you'll need to decrease your intensity a little to make it all the way through. Five extra minutes of aerobics is longer than you think! That means if you want to exercise longer, make sure your intensity is at a level that you can handle. Likewise, if you have less time and want to burn the same number of calories as you would for a longer duration, increase your intensity.

Type means the type of aerobic training that you are performing such as running, biking, or stepping. Type also refers to variety within an activity. For example, you can change your running program from flats to hills, or from sprints to light jogging. Use the FITT formula to adapt to the different *types* of exercise you're doing.

Training on Target

Keeping tabs on your heart rate when you exercise keeps your training in check. To monitor your exercise levels, use the target heart-rate chart on the following page. Count your pulse for ten seconds, starting with the number 1, then multiply by six. The chart, however, does it all for you. It's a good idea to check your pulse about five minutes into your program to see if you're in your training heart-rate range and then again after the most intense portion to see if you've maintained it. Check your pulse again after you've cooled down to see if your heart rate is lowering adequately.

Sample Target Heart-Rate Ranges
Beats per Minute & Ten-Second Pulse

	55%	85%
AGE	PULSE: 1 MIN (10 SEC)	PULSE: 1 MIN (10 SEC)
20	110 (18)	170 (28)
25	107 (18)	165 (27)
30	104 (17)	161 (26)
35	102 (17)	157 (26)
40	99 (16)	153 (25)
45	96 (16)	148 (24)
50	93 (16)	144 (24)
55	91 (15)	140 (23)
60	88 (15)	136 (22)

Equation: 220-age = MHR

MHR x Intensity % = 1 Minute Heart Rate

1 Minute Heart Rate divided by 6 = 10-Second Count

After a while, your body responses will tell you you're on target. Use the following perceived exertion chart to see if you're accurately listening to your body. Each number on the chart corresponds to heart-rate intensity. A good rule of thumb is that your heart-rate range should correspond to roughly ten times the number on the chart. For example, a "somewhat hard" perceived exertion would rate a "13," at which level a moderately fit person's heart rate should be around 130 beats a minute. Whichever method you use, *don't* just stop suddenly; this can cause dizziness and light-headedness because your blood carrying all that wonderful oxygen doesn't return as quickly to your heart and brain. Make sure that you keep moving for at least three to five minutes after you "stop" any vigorous exercise.

Borg Perceived-Exertion Chart

(G. A. V. Borg, "Psycophysical Bases of Physical Exertion," Medicine Science in Sports and Exercise. *Copyright 1982 by American College of Sports Medicine.)*

ORIGINAL 20-POINT SCALE

RATING	DESCRIPTION
6	
7	Very, very light
8	
9	Very light
10	
11	Fairly light
12	
13	Somewhat hard
14	
15	Hard
16	
17	Very hard
18	
19	Very, very hard
20	

What does it mean if your heart rate is too high? It means you should slow down a bit, particularly if you are feeling any nausea, dizziness, pain, or extreme muscle fatigue. These are danger signs of excess exercising. You should feel like you've worked out hard after finishing an exercise session, but you shouldn't feel *sick*. If your heart rate is too low, you can pick up the pace.

Dissipating Fat

People ask me all the time if they *have* to work out at lower intensities in order to burn fat. This is so deceptive. At rest, our bodies use fat as fuel, approximately at a 9-to-1 ratio of fat to carbohydrate. That isn't as good as it sounds because at rest you're burning hardly any calories and hardly anything multiplied by nine still isn't much. As workout intensities start to increase, however, so does the caloric expenditure. The ratio of carbohydrate-to-fat also changes because at higher (exhaustive) intensities, larger percentages of carbohydrate-to-fat are used. In essence, what your body really cares about at the end of a workout is the total amount of calories burned, not whether the calories were burned from carbohydrates or fats.

Think of it as withdrawing money from a bank. If I withdraw one hundred dollars in one-dollar bills, or in five twenty-dollar bills, it still amounts to one hundred dollars. It's the same with exercise. If you walk three miles and it takes you forty-five minutes, you'll burn approximately two hundred fifty calories. If you run three miles and it takes you twenty minutes, you will burn the same two hundred fifty calories. Walking is as good a fuel burner as running is; it's just that you have to walk for a longer period of time to get there. Fat is a fuel for exercise; if you move, it will burn.

Working out harder and faster won't necessarily speed up the process. You need to set a pace you can maintain. Exercising at too high a level might have a negative effect. When you're starting out, you need to work at lower intensities to build up gradually to higher levels. Remember the FITT principle. But beware, it's easy to get impatient and want to go faster well before our bodies are ready to respond to that kind of intensity. The myth to disregard here is that exercising at lower intensities is the *only* way to burn fat. The truth is, you need to work out at varied intensities, which includes both higher-level and lower-level workout sessions to challenge your body to change.

∽

*There is no thrill quite like doing something
you didn't know you could.*
—*Marjorie Holmes*

∽

For Starters

Be gentle with yourself, try and make exercise as enjoyable as possible. Experiment and look at ways to make it be like play. I know for myself, I can't ride a stationary bike unless I have something to distract me like something I've been wanting to read. This way, I can't wait to get back on the bike and finish another chapter! Then riding the bike becomes something I really enjoy doing, it entices my mind and my body to do it. You need to find ways that will make it more appealing to you so that you can be consistent with it.

Partner up with someone dependable. You need to have someone there that you can account to. Cher liked training with a partner. She's the only client I've ever had who really loved me exercising along with her. It really helped keep her motivated. Actually, Cher loved to exercise with as many of her close friends as possible. We always had a group. Her best friend and assistant, Paulette, was always working out with us; we even got "Bumper," her manager, exercising, which is really saying something!

Cross-train. There are many ways to be active. There's recreation and then there's working out. As you become more experienced in choosing the right form of exercise and the right intensities to work at, you will get to know when you need to recreate and when you need to work out. If you've been working out really intensely, you might need to just go for a walk or build sand castles on the beach. If you've been feeling really stressed, what you might need to do is run a few miles, then go to the gym, lift some heavy weights, and blow off some steam.

Learn to listen to your body. If you're tired and begin to overtrain, you could get injured. Make sure the exercises you're doing are in accordance with your goals. Backtrack a little, if you need to, and re-evaluate what your exercise choices are and make sure that you're comfortable.

The Overtraining Trap: Avoiding Injury

It's human nature to continue doing what feels good to you. Now that you're finally exercising, maybe you don't want to stop. However, there is a point when too much of a good thing turns into a trap. "More is better" doesn't necessarily apply to training. If what used to feel great is now a chore, or a flight of stairs is suddenly a breathless challenge, then you might be overdoing it.

The number one cause of overtraining is overuse; that is, too much of the same thing too often, without enough rest. The difficulty is identifying the problem because overtraining is easily masked by symptoms characteristic of other ailments that produce a similar "blah" response. Here's a list of overtraining symptoms. If you suffer from two or more of these for more than a few weeks, you might need to recover from burnout:

- sudden change in ability to exercise at the same intensity you've been at

- drastic weight loss in a very short period of time

- increase in resting heart rate

- breathless after workout of normal aerobic intensity

- loss of appetite or nausea after eating

- swelling or aching lymph glands in neck, underarm, or groin area

- anemia

- amenorrhea (loss of menstrual cycle)

- pain in muscles or joints

- muscle cramping at night

- difficulty sleeping

- edema (water retention)

- overuse injury like tendinitis or shin splints

- change of mood; irritable or depressed

How do you bust the blahs? Well, first you might need a break. I didn't say quit, just change your pace. Check your Life Circle and substitute some less strenuous activities to help get you back on track. Then vary your program, both in exercise and intensity levels; consider both rest and recreation as part of your program. You'll stay motivated, your body will love you, and you won't get injured.

Keli's Quick Fit Tips

1. Set goals . . . track progress . . . watch your success. Role models can help determine what and how to get inspired. Follow them!

2. Fitness is more a journey than a destination. Get comfortable and enjoy the ride!

3. Variety. Life isn't all apples and oranges. Cross-train, try out different activities. Find the ones that you enjoy: hiking, biking, walking, roller blading, outdoor stair climbing, dance classes, step classes, yoga, boxing, weight training. The choices are infinite!

4. Now make fitness a part of your lifestyle. Discipline is an action, not a feeling.

5. Don't diet!! Retrain old eating habits with new healthy ones for permanent fat loss. Learn to eat when you're hungry and stop before you're full. Eat regularly from a selection of low-fat, natural, simple, fresh, unprocessed foods.

6. Drink water . . . a minimum of eight glasses a day! Gain a healthy, glowing complexion, avoid premenstrual bloat.

7. In regard to pain, listen to your body. If it hurts, don't do it. There is a difference between an intense exercise and a dangerous one. Your body will tell you . . . all you have to do is listen!

8. Rest, let your body recover from your workouts, guilt-free! Let days off be for enriching your spirit and mind.

9. Think of it as fun and play . . . eager anticipation rather than dread. Find a way to let your workouts be rewarding. Be firm, yet

gentle and kind to yourself. Try exercising with your friends or a loved one, or let it be time for yourself.

10. Be patient, Rome wasn't built in a day. Persistence rather than perfection. Do it and keep at it; before you know it, you won't recognize yourself.

11. Let yourself glow; if you're exercising where there are mirrors and you're having a bad day, wear something that makes you feel beautiful. The mirror can be a friend and not just a foe.

∾

Enjoy your achievements as well as your plans.
—Max Ehrmann

∾

Real Aerobic Action

Remember at the beginning of this chapter I said, "Now the fun begins"? I meant it. Planning your program might seem complicated, but once you get started, the puzzle pieces will fit together. No need to cram; you have a lifetime of fitness to look forward to.

Let's put everything into perspective so that you can use all of your personal information wisely and then put it all to practice:

- In chapter 1, you set some immediate and long-term goals, noting your most important fitness goals in the activity questionnaire in this chapter.

- Your self-assessment from chapter 2 helped you evaluate your physical starting point as well as medical risk. Although your goals might be high, you still need to consider your physical condition.

You might have scored excellent on some assessments and lower on others. If you scored low or poor in the aerobic category, you'll want to start slowly and build your aerobic program gradually. If you scored low or poor in strength or flexibility, be sure to include at least two days of strength training and daily stretching to your plan.

- Check your risk profile, consider the activities you need to exercise, and change your lifestyle to reduce medical risk.

- Look at your activity questionnaire. What activities do you want to participate in to make fitness more fun? Choose your place, partners, and time of day.

- Look at your Life Circle. What activities do you want and need to round out your life?

- Organize a weekly fitness plan using the schedule at the end of this chapter. Don't overwhelm yourself and plan so far ahead that you lose sight and interest in the process. This might be setting yourself up for unattainable goals. Plan one week at a time, so you can change activities if you want for the next week. Allow flexibility for schedule changes and outside conflicts. Most important is to give yourself a schedule you can handle; this is about self-support, not self-sabotage.

Following is an example of how I set my clients on a program based on goals, assessments, and time schedules. Use this as a guide to help you plan your own program:

Leslie is thirty-one years old, five-foot-nine, and single. When she came to me, she weighed 165 pounds and her body fat was 25 percent. Leslie had no medical problems, although she was constantly under a lot of stress. She was exercising seven days a week, averaging one or two high-impact classes a day, although that caused her considerable knee pain. Her goals were to lose weight, increase flexibility, and increase her muscle tone and shape. Using the same tests detailed in this book, Leslie completed assessments, which showed she needed to increase her flexibility as well as gain stability in her thighs for her knees. Due to weak medial quadriceps, she had "smiley knees." When I calculated her BMR, she needed twenty-six hundred calories for maintenance of her current weight.

Leslie's Program:

Strength: Her program included weight training two times a week, sometimes three. She would take a body-sculpting class during weeks that she only weight-trained twice.

Cardiovascular: She began to vary her cardiovascular workout to include: high-impact aerobics only one to two times per week; the recumbent bike and upright bike; on alternating days, the Stairmaster, provided it didn't cause her pain; and some low-impact aerobics. She took up golf for her stress levels. We limited her aerobic activity to six hours a week with one full day off. However, we increased the intensity of her workouts and shortened the duration because she was exercising at low intensities with the intention of burning more fat, but her heart rate wasn't in her training zone.

Flexibility: We added daily stretches for her lower-body muscles, which were extremely tight, and also included some specific back and abdominal strength for stability. For her Life Circle, we added regular massage and made sure she took one full day to "putter" for stress.

Weight loss: I placed her on a twelve-hundred-calorie-a-day intake because she wanted fast results, but I also knew that she could eat sensibly and safely with this amount.

Nutrition: I had her drink more water and cut out sodas; modify her habitually excessive protein intake; substitute healthy activity for "stress-eating"; cut back alcohol consumption from two to three glasses per day to occasionally and replaced it with water or sparkling water.

Reassessment:

It's obvious by Leslie's results that this program was perfect for her. The added weight training stimulated her metabolism for fat loss by adding some muscle, and gave her a fabulously toned look. She didn't lose a lot on the scale but she lost a lot of fat. Her varied aerobic program plus the strength training alleviated her knee pain, plus gave her enough of a "stress release" so that she was free to do other leisurely activities. The change in her nutritional habits became easier as a result of reduced stress, which gave her the energy to handle her heavy workload.

Here's a chart summarizing the "before Leslie" and the "after Leslie":

Aug. 18—wt 165, body fat 25%   Oct. 1—wt 159, body fat 21%
Body fat: 47 lbs   Body fat: 35 lbs
                                                      Scale lost: 6 lbs
                                                      Body fat lost: 12 lbs

Beginning Measurements   **Ending Measurements**
Chest:............36.5"   Chest:............35.5"
Waist: ....30.5"   Waist: ....28.5"
Hips:..............40.5"   Hips:..............38.5"
Midthigh:......22.0"   Midthigh:......21.5"
Midcalf:.........15.0"   Midcalf:.........14.0"
Biceps: ....12.0"   Biceps: ....11.5"

Again, turn to the planner at the end of this chapter to design your personal weekly program. Before you start writing on it, be sure to photocopy as many pages as you think you might need for future use. Reassess this weekly to see if you want to change any activities or time and day of your workouts. Enjoy.

Activity Tips

Here are a few quick tidbits to remember for some basic aerobic activities. No matter how good exercise is, if it's done incorrectly, it can injure you. Form is so important; I can't tell you how much more you'll get out of your workout if you do it right. You'll triple your gains with a lot less effort.

Walking: You don't have to walk any particular way; we all have our own natural stride. When you walk, stay tall and long with head up and in line with the horizon, abdominals contracted, and shoulders relaxed. Keep your stride long and smooth, pushing through your heel to the ball of the foot as you step. Swing your arms naturally in opposition. For a more vigorous walk, keep your elbows bent at a 90-degree angle and pump your arms forward and back without twisting your shoulders side to side, so your forward arm reaches breastbone height with each swing. Lean slightly forward from the lower body—not your waist—as if you want to get somewhere (maybe a great sale!).

Running: Although running or jogging is a natural skill like walking, some people prefer walking quickly to running. If you like to run, keep your stride smooth; don't worry so much about speed. Keep your body fairly upright with your back in a neutral position with your head up; look about five paces ahead of your step. Your arms should be close to your waist so your elbows are at a 90-degree angle with your forearms parallel to the ground. Don't clench your fingers; keep them loose. Your arms should swing rhythmically forward and back, not side to side.

Stationary bikes: First things first: Adjust the seat so you can reach the pedals comfortably. When pedaling, you should be able to straighten your legs with only a slight bend to your knees. This would be the same for a mountain bike or a regular touring bike if you're street riding. Place your feet through the foot straps so the arch and ball of the foot push down and through the pedal for the most power. Now, sit up straight, no slouching, and hold on to the handlebars. One of the biggest mistakes people make is leaning forward on the handlebars.

Even if you want to read or watch TV, sit up with your back straight so your abdominals have to work. Set your program, level, and time as you begin to pedal. Push with even strokes that set a cadence. If you're outdoors, remember to watch the terrain and the traffic.

Stairmasters: I get on the warpath when I watch people on a stairclimber, mainly because I know they're wasting their time and might injure themselves. Do not, I repeat, do not lean on the handles so your derriere sticks out behind you and step as fast as you can on your toes!!! Whew, that's off my chest. If you're going to stair climb, keep your body straight so your back is in a neutral position. That means your tailbone points downward to the floor, not behind you like a tail. Hold on to the support bars *with* your thumbs forward so palms face inward, not outward. Keep as much of your foot on the pedal as possible and push downward with each step so your foot *remains in contact* with the pedal. Stair climbing can give you a great aerobic workout, but you need to set yourself up to step right.

Let me close this part with some favorite words of wisdom:

FITNESS
Don't be afraid to work hard,
Don't be afraid to fail,
Don't be afraid to be fit, to be strong . . .
Don't be afraid to dream big dreams,
Don't be afraid to define your own life—never give
anyone else the power to define your life,
Don't be afraid to love each other,
You can't reach to others if you don't fundamentally
love yourself, and that's what fitness is all about . . .
—Dr. James Rippe

Notes

Notes

Notes

Notes

Notes

FIVE

Warm-Up

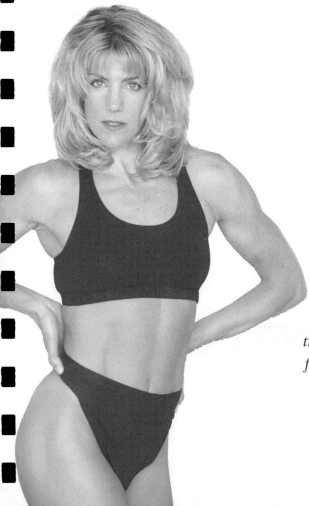

ACTING AS IF . . .
*You've got to get up every
morning with a smile on
your face, and show the
world all the love in your
heart. Then people gonna
treat you better; you're gonna
find, yes you will, that you're
as beautiful as you feel.*
—Carol King

Now you've set up your realistic fitness goals and you're ready to just *go*! Before you do, however, just hang on a minute . . . *you've got to warm up*!

Gradually easing into your daily program when your body feels more prepared isn't holding back. It's smart. There are major benefits associated with warming up, the most important being a better workout with less stress. Although there isn't any exact research which guarantees that a workout with a warm-up will prevent injury, it's a well-accepted fact that warming up with low-level activity, followed by some mild stretching, will certainly enhance your overall effort.

I find that warming up is essential for my motivation. It's the time I use to step out of where I've been and into where I'm going, both mentally and physically. I know the extra five or so minutes a day spent before your workout is well worth it.

Why Warm Up?

I don't know about you, but I sure can be stiff first thing in the morning (and it always feels like I'm about ten years older). But once I'm up and about, I'll loosen up and feel better. Warming up for the day is similar to warming up for exercise. The more you move, the better you'll feel. It seems that if you've been up and about all day, this would be sufficient preparation, but getting ready for exercise requires a little more than walking from the computer to the conference room . . . even if you are walking at a pretty quick pace.

One client who trained with me in the evening would often feel tired by the time she came in, but she knew that once she got into her warm-up, her energy would start to kick in. Once that happened, she would then fly through her workout, feeling so much better and energized by the end of it. She was always so surprised how it worked like that—that she could start off with no energy and end up with so much. I attribute her change in energy partly to the fact that her body was letting go of all her pent-up stress and tension while she warmed up. This woman lost thirty-eight pounds and dropped four dress sizes over a period of a year and a half. She accomplished this without dieting, but just by working out and making some simple changes in her dietary habits.

What are you waiting for?

Prior to beginning any exercise program, whatever it is, it's imperative to first do some type of active movement that will get you ready for more vigorous exercise. You do this by gradually increasing your heart rate, blood flow, and body temperature. When your muscles and connective tissue are "warm," they're more pliable, thus making them less susceptible to tearing. The same is true for your joints. When you move, your joints secrete a fluid—synovia—that lubricates them, so they'll feel loose and relaxed, making it easier to increase both your exercise intensity and range of motion.

What Is a Warm-up?

Better yet, what constitutes a warm-up? For starters, I recommend either (1) a brisk walk while swinging your arms naturally; (2) pedaling on the lowest level of a stationary cycle; or (3) simply marching in place while doing some arm circles. Your goal is twofold: to ensure that enough blood gets pumped to the heart and to increase blood flow to the entire body. Otherwise, exercise—even at lower intensities—can be uncomfortable. *The key to a good warm-up is getting active for at least five minutes, maybe longer, depending on what type of exercise routine you'll be doing and how your body feels. You know you're warmed up when you feel ready to pick up a more vigorous pace.*

Once you're mildly warmed up—you might even have broken a light sweat—do some easy stretching to further prepare the connective tissue (ligaments and tendons) for whatever activity you've chosen. Stretch only to the point of mild tension and hold each stretch for about thirty seconds. Give special attention to muscles you're going to work that day. My ten-step stretch plan explained in this chapter will dramatically enhance your total-body program, which can be geared toward virtually any sport or activity.

Overstretching Your Limits

Warming up isn't about increasing muscle flexibility, although it's important to include some stretching as part of the whole package. Just know, however, that stretching and warming up are not the same. You don't want to stretch a cold muscle, so make sure you first do some limbering movements, such as those previously mentioned. Listen to your body and don't overstretch. Otherwise, you might be defeating your purpose.

When you stretch too far, you cause your muscles to respond in a way similar to that of a rubber band when it's overstretched. A rubber band will only stretch so far before it tries to spring back to its original shape. Placing too much tension on your muscles can cause what's called the stretch reflex, which is your body's natural response to let you know you've gone too far. This causes your muscles to contract, rather than elongate and relax. So keep your stretching gentle. Stretching should feel good, not painful. Forget the "no-pain, no-gain" maxim for the time being.

Create Mental Pictures

If the weather is cold or you're exercising earlier than usual in the day, it might take you a little longer to warm up. Don't be hard on yourself. Enjoy this time, because it's getting you ready mentally, too.

Many times my clients come rushing in for a workout and want to jump right in without a warm-up. Not good. I encourage them to take the extra five minutes needed to get their blood flowing and become mentally ready. A warm-up is just as important psychologically as it is physically.

When my clients can get their minds as well as their bodies present, all of their attention is focused on themselves and their workout, as it should be. Getting them to take a moment to breathe, stretch, and then visualize what they want to accomplish enables them to get more out of the workout. When you're not mentally focused, you're more apt to hurt yourself or end up feeling like your workout was inadequate. Use your warm-up time to reaffirm your goals—to mentally rehearse. Imagine what a great workout you're about to have, and let your ultimate motivator be the knowledge of how great you'll feel when you've finished.

Taking a moment to take it easy is being a friend to yourself.
—Heart Warmers

Warm-up Do's

- Include a full-body warm-up, even if you're isolating a body part.
- Warm up for a minimum of five to ten minutes, gradually increasing intensity.
- Do rhythmic limbering movements prior to static stretching.
- Use full range of motion without locking your joints.
- Think about your movement and how your body feels while you're doing it.
- Stretch without bouncing, holding each stretch to the point of mild tension.
- Mentally rehearse, focus, and motivate yourself.

My Ten-Step Stretch Plan

Directions: Do the following stretches in the order shown. Hold each stretch for about thirty seconds without bouncing.

1   HAMSTRING STRETCH

Muscles stretched: rear of thigh (hamstrings) and buttocks (gluteus maximus)

Setup

1. Stand erect with feet hip-width apart and place one foot two to three inches in front of the other, with the toes of your front foot lifted.
2. Place hands on front of thighs for support.

Action

1. Keep front leg straight with toes lifted and bend other knee to "sit" directly backward, while keeping spine erect.
2. Place body weight on support leg so that your torso is leaning at about a 45-degree angle, with your head, neck, and spine aligned.
3. Keep front toes lifted to help keep body weight toward rear heel of support leg.
4. As you lean back, you'll feel a stretch in the rear of your front leg, which is still straight.
5. Straighten support leg to stand upright, then change legs to stretch other side.

Training tips

1. Keep spine straight; do not round the back as you go into the stretch.
2. To protect knees, keep body weight toward heel of support leg.
3. Bend from the hips and knees so your entire torso leans; keep chest lifted without bending from the waist.
4. Keep feet hip-width apart for better balance.

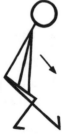

Hamstring Stretch Modification

1. If balance is difficult, do this same exercise while holding on to the back of a chair or other sturdy support.

2   CALF STRETCH

Muscles stretched: calves (gastronemius), hip flexors (iliopsoas)

Setup

1. Facing a wall, stand at arm's length from the wall and place one foot in front of the other, with toes pointing forward about hip-width apart.
2. Place hands on the wall with elbows slightly bent, about shoulder-width apart.
3. Adjust legs so they're separated enough so that when you bend your front knee, it stays in line with your ankle.
4. Contract abdominals and keep your tailbone down.

Action

1. Bend front knee and press hips forward, keeping your back leg straight with heel on the floor.
2. Make sure spine remains straight and rib cage lifted, with shoulders and hips square.

Training tips

1. To stretch the calf, your back heel must remain on the floor with toes pointing forward, as if your back foot were on a balance beam.
2. Keep front foot in line with ankle.
3. Press forward from the hip without arching back.

Modification

1. If you have the tendency to arch your back, stand a little closer to the wall and place your entire forearm on it rather than just your hands.

3 QUADRICEPS STRETCH

Muscles stretched: front of thigh (quadriceps), hip flexors (iliopsoas)

Setup

1. Facing a wall, stand at arm's length from the wall with feet hip-width apart, knees slightly bent, and pelvis in neutral alignment, with tailbone pointing down and abdominals contracted.
2. Place one hand on wall for support.

Action

1. Bend one knee, bringing heel up toward buttocks, and grasp front of the ankle with hand on same side, keeping support knee relaxed to maintain alignment.
2. Hold your ankle so both knees are close together and the bent knee points to the floor, so you feel a stretch in the front of the hip and thigh of the bent leg.
3. Keep back in a neutral position without arching or leaning forward; keep head up and abdominals contracted.

Training tips

1. Keep shoulders and hips square.
2. Keep knees close together.
3. Avoid pulling heel to buttocks; this is a mild stretch.

Modification

1. If you cannot hold ankle without arching, stand so hips and pelvis are braced against the wall and do the same stretch.

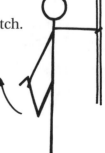

4 HIP FLEXOR STRETCH

Muscles stretched: hip flexors (iliopsoas)

Setup
1. Stand in a staggered lunge position with one foot in front of the other, both knees bent to a 90-degree angle so front knee is over ankle and rear knee points to the floor with rear heel lifted.
2. Place hands on hips for support.
3. Contract abdominals so spine is erect with tailbone pointing down.

Action
1. Maintain bent-knee position of the legs; tighten buttocks and tilt pelvis forward until you feel a stretch in the front of the hip of your rear leg.

Training tips
1. This is a small movement; don't overtilt pelvis.
2. As you tilt, the front of the hip should "flatten"; feel leg lengthen.

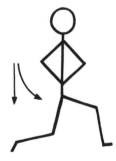

5 CHEST STRETCH

Muscles stretched: chest (pectoralis major) and front of shoulders (anterior deltoid)

Setup
1. Stand in the center of an open doorway, feet in a lunge position and one foot in front of the other, with abdominals contracted and tailbone pointing down.
2. Place one forearm on the wall just outside the doorjamb with elbow at shoulder height.

Action
1. Maintain body position and gently lean forward, pressing through the chest until you feel a stretch on your chest.

Training tips
1. Lean slightly forward; stay upright.
2. As you lean, press against the wall with forearm for more of a stretch.
3. Keep shoulder and arm bent at a 90-degree angle.

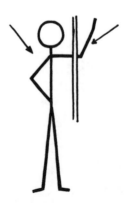

6 BACK STRETCH

Muscles stretched: upper, middle, and lower back (trapezius, rhomboids, latissimus dorsi, erector spinae), rear and middle shoulders (medial and posterior), and buttocks (gluteus maximus)

Setup
1. Stand and face a sturdy support (such as a pole, a door, or a sink counter), with feet a little wider than hip-width apart, knees slightly bent, with abdominals contracted and tailbone pointing down.
2. Extend both arms in front of you at chest height and grasp the support with both hands, shoulders down and back.

Action
1. Bend knees and tuck tailbone under as you sit back so your body weight is toward your heels, allowing your back to round like the letter C, and open your shoulder blades.
2. Drop chin so that head and neck follow the natural curve of spine as you stretch.
3. Pull back away from support to increase stretch.

Training tips
1. Keep abdominals contracted, so back can round and stretch.
2. Don't "dive" forward; the movement should feel like you're sinking down and back into the floor, with knees still in line with ankles.

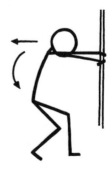

7   CHEST STRETCH

Muscles stretched: chest (pectoralis major), front of shoulders (anterior deltoid), and front of upper arm (biceps)

Setup

1. Stand with feet about hip-width apart, knees bent, and tailbone pointing down toward the floor.
2. Hold arms behind you, hands close to buttocks, with elbows slightly bent and one palm inside the other.
3. Contract abdominals, press shoulder blades down and together to relax shoulders.

Action

1. Maintain body position and gently lift arms away from buttocks until you feel a stretch across chest and shoulders.

Training tips

1. Don't lean backward as you stretch; maintain an upright posture.
2. Keep body weight balanced over the center of your arches.
3. Lift gently, keeping shoulders back and down.

Modification

1. Hold a towel or resistance tube in each hand behind you if your shoulders are tight.

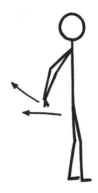

8   SIDE STRETCH

Muscles stretched: middle back (latissimus dorsi), sides of torso (obliques)

Setup

1. Stand with legs wider than shoulder-width apart, feet turned out slightly, with one knee bent to a 90-degree angle, the other leg straight.
2. Contract abdominals and lift rib cage.
3. Place one hand on thigh of bent knee for support and extend the opposite arm in the air, close to your ear.

Action

1. Maintain lower-body position and slowly lean toward bent leg so arm above head and straight leg form a diagonal line and you feel a stretch in the side of your torso.

Training tips

1. Don't lean so far sideways that you throw your hip out to the side and lose alignment.
2. Avoid slouching or bending the torso sideways; it is definitely a full body lean and upward reach.
3. Keep rib cage lifted and abdominals contracted.

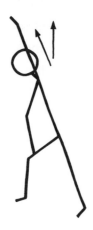

9 OVERHEAD STRETCH

Muscles stretched: rear of upper arm (triceps)

Setup
1. Stand with feet hip-width apart, knees slightly bent, and tailbone pointing down.
2. Bend one elbow, placing hand on your shoulder close to your neck.
3. Place opposite hand underneath elbow.

Action
1. Keep hand on shoulder and use support hand to lift arm overhead until elbow points to the ceiling and you feel a stretch on the rear of your upper arm.
2. Keep shoulders relaxed.

Training tips
1. Keep spine straight and in neutral position, with abdominals contracted as you lift arm overhead.
2. Look straight ahead, shoulders down.

Modification
1. For inflexible shoulders and triceps, hold a towel over your shoulder and down your back with elbow pointed to the ceiling. With the opposite hand behind your back and close to waist, pull downward on other end of the towel.

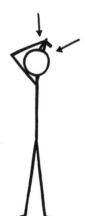

10 SIDE-TO-SIDE STRETCH

Muscles stretched: neck (levator scapula), upper back muscles (trapezius)

Setup
1. Stand erect with feet hip-width apart, knees bent, and pelvis in good alignment, with arms relaxed by your sides.
2. Contract abdominals, drop shoulders down and back, and look straight ahead.

Action
1. Slowly bring one ear toward shoulder, keeping shoulders down and maintaining body alignment, while you elongate your neck muscles.

Training tips
1. Drop ear to shoulder; don't lift shoulder toward ear.
2. Maintain a comfortable, relaxed stance.
3. If you prefer, close your eyes as you stretch.

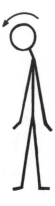

Notes

Notes

Notes

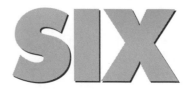

SIX

Strength-Training Concepts

STRENGTH

The quality or state of being strong: physical power. It is the power of resisting strain or force, a degree of potency of concentration.

—Random House Dictionary

Why strength train? When I first started strength training ten years ago in that little gym back in Australia, I had no clue how pushing some weight around would completely change my body and my life. All I knew was that I was heavy and needed to exercise—what did I have to lose by trying? Well, as I discovered, I lost a whole lot of fat and increased more than just muscle mass; I gained back my health and self-respect.

The physiological and psychological benefits of strength training are tremendous. You don't have to spend an enormous amount of time in the gym to obtain toned, strong muscles. Obviously, if you want to be more "buff," you'll train harder and longer. But for positive health gains, two to three times a week is adequate. Here's what you can expect from a moderate weekly training program:

1. Strong bones, which are more dense; this is crucial to help prevent the development of osteoporosis in women.

2. Better posture because your muscles are balanced; this improves the overall integrity and protection of the spine.

3. Daily activities and sports will be easier to perform.

4. Muscle tone and definition will improve, along with improved shape, size, and symmetry.

5. Strength training adds more muscle, increasing your body's energy requirements. We therefore burn calories at a higher rate, even at rest.

6. Reduction in body fat because of the increased number of calories used.

7. Increased coordination and neuromuscular function; once you've been training, you'll use more muscle fiber per muscle contraction than an untrained person will.

8. If you're an athlete, strength training can help improve power, flexibility, and agility.

9. You'll feel stronger, more confident, and operate with a higher level of self-esteem.

10. Reduction in the risk of injury because your muscles and connective tissue are stronger.

These changes don't occur at the same time or overnight, but if you're diligent with your program, you certainly can expect to see significant differences in both your body and how you feel in a relatively short period of time.

Strength Training for Health

Most of my clients come to me with a better body in mind, first and foremost. Improving their health is usually not even on the list. I think people sometimes "settle" for the way they feel because they never realized they had viable options. Anita, my sixty-four-year-old client, had high blood pressure when we started. She doesn't have high blood pressure now! Even with medication, her blood pressure was too high, and now it's a little below normal. Her doctor is considering taking her off the medication altogether because she has controlled the condition with consistent aerobics and weight training.

Says Anita, "I had never worked out before. Now, I don't get up like older people who take a while to stand up, plus I look good. I don't have any of the symptoms attributed to old age."

In the past, individuals with high blood pressure were advised to stay away from weight training because it was thought to exacerbate the problem. It's only been recently that new studies have shown that weight training actually can assist in lowering blood pressure.

I had another client, Peter, who I consider one of my true success stories. Prior to our working together, he endured major back surgery. When he came to me, he had been bedridden since surgery and couldn't walk. Today, he weight trains and even gardens.

"Over the last two years, I'm impressed with my results in terms of shape and weight," Peter said. "My recovery has been complete, and friends are amazed that I could go so quickly from bed to being in excellent shape."

I'm going to make weight training for you as "user-friendly" as possible, so you, too, can get started today, whether you've done it before or not.

Strength-Training Principles

Overload

One of the key components of strength training is that it *overloads* your muscles. If you want your body to change, you need to train it just a little harder than it's used to. If your program is comfortable, and you can get through all the reps and sets with very little effort, you're not placing enough overload on your muscles to stress them.

The best way to overload is with progressive resistance. This is a systematic method of increasing your weight each time the exercises get easier or are no longer challenging. Increasing weight in this way creates *intensity* that forces muscles to change. We can create a similar intensity by manipulating other variables of overload: number of reps and/or sets, exercise order and selection, and speed.

The most frequent thing I've seen in watching people train is they underload. They do way too many reps, but never reach the point of fatigue or muscle failure. You'd be surprised how strong women can get without getting big. My women frequently do twenty-pound dumbbell flys to train their chest muscles, while women next to them will be doing seven-pound flys. Seven pounds! The chest is a large, strong muscle group. Seven pounds won't overload regularly trained pecs.

I always have to remind my new women clients that they will *not* get *big* from strength training by lifting heavy weights; they'll get strong. I know many women who won't strength train because they're terrified of looking like Attila the Hun. Women will say to me, "Oh, I don't want to get my legs big." Don't worry. Factors such as your genetics and how your body responds are more influential when it comes to the benefits of weight lifting.

You know, I can lunge all day long (lunges are *great* exercises for legs!), but the moment I substitute in a leg press, my legs thicken up, so I know it's not the right exercise for *me*. Yet my client, Marjorie, can leg press, and her legs look fantastic. The point is, I'm talking about *shape*, not *size*. Different exercises will have different effects on your muscles. If you're a woman, you *cannot* get really big because you aren't genetically programmed the same way a man is; we have much less testosterone as part of our hormonal balance.

The way someone responds to an exercise is genetics, too. Marjorie's body is programmed to respond to certain movements differently than my body does. Here's the best bit: If your muscles grow into a certain shape, and you don't like that shape, it's *reversible!* I just love that!!

By focusing on your body and how you can redefine it or redesign it, you can constantly keep fine-tuning your program to keep modifying the specific response. The longer you train, the more specific the response you can create and maintain! That's incredibly motivating, especially once you come to understand and experience this control. In chapter 7, I describe five different programs in great detail to help you achieve this.

Choosing a Starting Weight

Unfortunately, I don't have any simple formula to give you. You'll need to choose the amount of weight for each exercise by trial and error, based on your goals. You need to predetermine if you want to train for strength or endurance because the number of repetitions and amount of weight you use are interrelated.

Since each person begins training at different initial strength levels, the amount of weight that person can lift varies extremely from one individual to another. Also, strength varies from muscle group to muscle group, so there isn't a set weight you would be starting with for every body part.

Here's one method: For each exercise, choose an amount of weight you "believe" you can handle and complete at least eight repetitions, but not more than fifteen. If you can accomplish this easily, you need more weight. If you can't, find a weight that you can. One more thing: Don't choose weight so heavy that you can only complete some of the exercises. Challenge your muscles to near maximum effort with each exercise. Use progressive resistance to keep increasing the weight as you improve.

Reps and Sets

Besides weight, you can change the number of reps and sets to create exercise intensity. A set is made up of a designated amount of repetitions, which is dependent upon the amount of weight that you're using. In general, you'll do less reps with heavier weight, though the *number of sets* may stay the same; the reverse would be true of less weight, you'd do more reps.

Although increasing muscle endurance is important, I really believe it's important to train specifically for strength improvements. For a moderate program, you'll need to do at least two to three sets of anywhere between eight and twelve repetitions. More reps than twelve per set becomes more endurance-oriented.

Exercise Selection

Many of my clients complain about specific body parts they want to change, such as buttocks or abdominals. I'm sure if I let them, they'd do buttocks exercises all day! You need to consider your body as a whole. To maintain posture, muscle balance, and strength, you need to include at least one exercise for every major muscle. That's only twelve exercises; I've done that for you in chapter 7 in the introductory program. Equally important is training *opposing* muscle groups, since your muscles work in pairs. This will give you a symmetrical, well-proportioned body.

Exercise Order

In general, work your largest muscles first, such as your legs or back, especially if you're using heavier weights. Large-muscle-group exercises tend to be more multimuscle anyway, so your smaller groups, such as the deltoids or biceps, get a good warm-up for when you want to isolate them later in your workout. If you start with your smaller muscles, they'll fatigue too quickly and not be of much help with larger movements.

Range of Motion and Speed

I don't know if you've ever tried to "pump" a twenty-five-pound dumbbell for biceps curls, but I wouldn't advise it for biceps—or any other muscle group for that matter! To get the full benefit of your training, work through the full range of motion for each exercise *slowly*. This puts the most tension on the muscle, increasing the force with a lower rate of injury. This is *so* important!! You'll be able to apply so much more resistance and control to your movements if you do. I generally recommend two seconds on the upward phase of the movement and four seconds on the downward or stretching phase.

Rest

Rest is important as part of your workout and in between workouts. Resting between sets allows your muscles to recover from the temporary fatigue caused by the set you just did. However, if you're waiting more than two minutes in between sets, you're wasting your time! If you're spending two hours in the gym, you're definitely sitting around. It's about tension and the building up of that tension that creates the overload so necessary for any results. If you're resting for too long, the tension levels decrease and you'll not stimulate the muscles nearly as well. The only time I would ever recommend longer than a one- to one-and-a-half-minute break is if you are power lifting with very heavy weight.

As you decrease the amount of rest between sets and/or exercises, the intensity of your training increases. I like to reduce rest periods as a way of adding variety to training, or restimulating the body if it's not continuing to change. In chapter 7, I talk about supersetting programs, in which you don't rest at all in between exercises. These programs are designed to keep going to get full benefit. By the time you've set up the exercise and move on, you've had adequate rest to just keep going.

The other rest time to have in your workout is *rest days.* Your body needs time to recover from training. If you're doing all of your exercises on the same day, make sure you allow at least one to two days of rest in between. If you're splitting your workout by body parts, the same would apply. For example, if you're doing upper body two days a week and lower two days a week, or back, biceps, and legs on one day, and chest, shoulders, and triceps on another, you need to rest at least one day before you repeat those body parts. This is sensible training.

Fatigue vs. Failure

Here's the truth about weight training: The last two reps or so aren't supposed to be comfortable; they should be very challenging, and you should feel your muscles really working to complete the repetitions. This is a good thing; this is muscle fatigue. You need to achieve this point to stimulate muscle change. If you tried to do another rep and couldn't even lift the weight, this is muscle failure. When you're exercising alone, it's very difficult to work yourself to failure. And it can be risky if you're using maximum effort and not maintaining good form. However, by the last few reps, you should be working very hard: it should be a great effort, with you pushing pretty close *to* maximum effort, but you can still complete the rep.

Here's a suggestion: If you want to get a little bit more from the set, after completing your twelfth or fifteenth rep without resting, reduce the weight by about ten or fifteen pounds, so that you can do another six to eight reps. And then if you're in the mood to work *really* hard, you can do it a second time. I highly recommend this "drop set" type of training. It's safe, you'll see good results, see your body really change, and you'll see your strength levels really go up.

If you have a partner, of course, you can do a lot of other things. They can assist and spot you so that you can get that extra rep in that you couldn't do alone.

Breathing

I used to think that breathing was the most natural process—who had to be taught how to breathe? When I first started training, I'd catch myself forgetting to breathe at all while I concentrated to lift more weight. As I became accustomed to weight training, breathing naturally came easier.

Breathing naturally is the key—an inhale and exhale with every repetition. In general, exhale with the most resistive part of the exercise, and inhale as you release. This will maintain your normal breathing pattern so you don't experience any light-headedness or dizziness sometimes associated with holding your breath or overbreathing.

Consistency

One of the best explanations of the value of consistency came from my client, Marjorie, when she was pregnant: "When you're consistent, your weight is not on a roller coaster; you can maintain a sense of control.

"If you work out on a consistent basis, not even rigorously, you can still keep a consistent body look and fitness level," Marjorie said. "If you exercise three times a week and put in even an hour of good, solid focused time each time, that can be just as effective as if you come in five times a week once a month.

"A theme-park, roller-coaster body gets overtrained, and then rebels and demands cotton candy, and then you wind up looking all soft and buttery. Then it takes a while to even get back on the roller coaster, longer to get in shape, and then you're off it again, never having a chance to catch up. It's a vicious cycle. Like running on a hamster wheel, you never get a chance to get caught up."

What got Marjorie off the hamster wheel was working out when she was pregnant. Although she was working hard, she still got bigger every day, and the experience taught her to have patience with her body. She said, "I had to control my breathing more and become more internalized about the workout in all ways. When you're pregnant, you're forced to relax through your workout. You don't have the choice to grunt."

It made Marjorie realize you can relax through a workout and be mentally calm, and still receive the effects of being strong: "I was still increasing the weights, even though I wasn't pushing excessively or straining," she said.

Marjorie learned during the pregnancy that even a little bit of working out is better than doing nothing, because working out again after nine months of doing nothing would be twice as difficult. Besides, the *results* become internalized as well. You're working out for your baby, and getting more oxygen to her; she's getting a workout, you're getting a workout, and the ultimate result is giving birth.

"That's the ultimate exercise—learning to breathe all the way through and then passing this child through your body," Marjorie said.

"It's like the final marathon. You have to train for it. Eating bonbons isn't going to cut it."

Hannah was born strong and very healthy—six pounds, twelve ounces, and twenty inches long—and Marjorie gained only twenty-six pounds. This was accomplished with the moderate exercise that we did three or four times a week, while she ate what she wanted. Afterward, the weight came off an awful lot easier because of training *consistently* through the pregnancy. "It was as though my muscles had memory," she said.

∾

There is nothing permanent except change.
—Heraclitus

∾

Peaked-Out Performance

If your workout has come to a standstill, you might have hit a plateau. You'll know, because you'll get to a point where you stop making improvements. You'll have made significant gains, then you'll make slower gains, then you won't make any gains. You'll simply grind to a halt. The same exercises don't quite create the same overload, your body stops changing, and you don't feel that "good soreness" anymore.

Over the years I've noticed that plateaus precede injury. People will plateau and then they'll keep doing the same exercises, which can lead to overuse of those muscles. Before you know it, there's an injury. But if you cross-train and keep changing the stimuli in your program, then you won't necessarily hit any plateau, or at least hit one long enough that you become stale or even injured.

To avoid plateaus in the first place, I start my clients on a simple, basic strength regime and build them up to where they are training at their most advanced levels. The length of time it will take depends on where they started, how regularly they train, and their mentality. After they reach very advanced levels of training and start to plateau with supersets, I then encourage them to switch to circuit training for a couple of weeks and do more high-volume, low-intensity, endurance-based exercise to stimulate change. If you're lifting heavy weights with low repetitions, you'll find going to a circuit actually very challenging.

Apart from injury, plateauing should be one of the most avoidable things in fitness training. You don't ever have to reach a point of not improving the body. It's natural to hit the leveling-off period; you just don't have to stay there. It's like a little message the body sends that says, "Now it's time to change the program!" If you train smart, you won't plateau, or if you do, it will be temporary.

Training Tailor Fit

To repeat for the sake of emphasis, the ultimate challenge in keeping your workouts fresh and stimulating and mentally stimulating is *variation*. It's so simple and such great fun to experiment. You can create a completely different stimulus for a muscle group just by changing the type of bar that you use for the same exercise; this is particularly true for those of you who are more experienced. For people just starting out, it's more important to develop smooth form. But for those in advanced training, there's no reason the routine can't be slightly varied almost every time. In fact, that's what I do with my more advanced clients, although everyone has basic staples.

If a certain exercise really works for a certain area of the client's hip or back, for example, then I'll keep him or her on that exercise and maybe vary the grip a little bit. But that will be one exercise that person will do regularly. I'll vary the order in which he or she does it, and I'll vary the other exercises working the same part of the body, but that particular exercise will remain.

Weight Training for Weight Loss

When an overweight person comes to me, the first thing I do is put her on a weight-training program in addition to cardiovascular work. The amount of calories you burn in a workout isn't really that high. What counts is the total response—how your metabolism burns calories when you're outside the gym, walking around the office, or sitting at your desk . . . even when you're asleep. When you have more muscle mass, you have a faster metabolism.

Think about it like this: If you have a 1.3-liter engine and you're idling or accelerating, you don't use much fuel. You're pretty fuel-efficient. But if you have a V-8, all of a sudden, it's a different story. And if you have a fuel-injected V-8, then you are one fuel-hungry piece of machinery! Well, weight training gives you the opportunity to exchange your 1.3-liter engine for a V-8. You're going to be using more fuel when you're sitting watching TV—your whole metabolism is going to be elevated! I now eat a good twenty-five hundred to three thousand calories a day just to maintain my body weight because my metabolism is so much higher. When we started doing both cardiovascular and strength training for Cher, we saw a significant change in her body.

One of my favorite studies—a strength-research study conducted by Wayne Wescott, author of *Be Strong: Strength Training for Muscular Fitness for Men and Women*—compares exercisers who only participated in aerobic exercise three times a week for thirty minutes with exercisers who also exercised three times a week, but split the same thirty minutes into fifteen minutes of cardiovascular work and fifteen minutes of strengthening. Guess what? The people who only did aerobics lost only four pounds of fat, compared to the combo group that lost *ten* pounds of fat, plus gained some muscle mass! The weight-loss formula for the nineties isn't about dieting and running. To change your body, to lose fat, and/or to increase calories burned, add strength training to your program.

Right on Focus

I think the true psychology behind successful training is your focus during the set. Stress reduction is one of the benefits of a regular exercise program; there are two different components in that—tuning in and tuning out. There's a type of exercise that's a no-brainer. You don't think, you don't focus. You put yourself on autopilot and off you go, like when you ride a bicycle and read a book. That's perfectly valid and very important, if it fits your needs at the time.

But weight training is not an exercise with which you can do that. Weight training requires absolute, 100-percent concentration. Focus on how your body feels during the exercise. Focus on the muscle you're working, how it stretches and contracts, the blood building up in the muscle, and the effect all this intensity has on the contraction; then you picture the contraction. You find the mirror or a spot on the ceiling, and you focus on that. It's very important, and it's just as much of a stress release as the tune-out because you're not focusing on all the daily craziness.

When I work with women clients, I find I have a very hard time getting them to be aggressive enough with the weights. Strength training requires a certain amount of aggression, which I don't think is a bad thing. It's a very healthy emotion to express in the right situation; weight training can be a very appropriate place to release that emotion. Aggressive doesn't mean fast, either. It means being emotionally aggressive with it to push through those final difficult reps. That's when recognizable body changes happen fastest.

One of Susan Dey's goals when she first started with me was to relieve the incredible amount of pressure she has on a daily basis. She told me once, "Anger and frustration are held in our bodies; when you work out, you work through that. Stress isn't something that just goes in your brain, where you're carrying the load. It goes into your cells as physical reaction to stress. Exercise is the only thing for me that cleans my body of these unwanted emotions, the way a lizard sheds its skin.

It feels like my muscles are working past the stress and toxins created by the stress because I breathe differently; oxygen is going in, my body is moving, which is shaking the stress."

Being physically stronger makes you mentally and emotionally able to overcome life's hurdles. Lifting helps me push those personal blocks and problems away from me. It's actually incredibly therapeutic. If you're bench pressing, and you're pushing and you're pushing, you learn to push through those last few reps, with the same strength that helps you to overcome outside pressures. It applies to your everyday life. When my life's circumstances become difficult, I head straight to the weight room.

Women in our culture are taught to *not* stand up for themselves, to be passive, to yield. And one thing I like about weight training is the inner strength it takes to say, "I'm not going to yield to this! I'm going to do these last few reps!" Learning to assert yourself to go through those last three reps helps you to ask for what you need, and to speak up with an opinion. I've seen it help myself as well as my clients learn to be truly assertive. Weight training teaches a physical and mental assertiveness that can be taken out into the world.

Notes

Notes

Notes

SEVEN

Program Design

JOURNEY

*It's good to have an end
to journey toward;
but it is the journey that
matters in the end.*
—Ursula K. Leguin

hope you're ready to start training because that's what this chapter is all about. I'm going to walk you through the four programs I've designed for you. By the time you get to program five, you should be ready to design your own.

I'm a firm believer in sensible strength training. The exercises I've chosen are not only my favorites, but they also work each muscle most specifically to induce strength gains and change body shape. I have seen fantastic results with my clients, whether they use program 1 or program 3; it's a matter of what you're ready for.

Strength training is steeped deeply in tradition and sometimes myth. Every serious bodybuilder believes in his or her own set formula to train by, sometimes ignoring safety, form, and technique for the sake of size. I can assure you, while I've included *traditional* and popular exercises, this is a straightforward, well-rounded, and broad *approach* to training. You don't have to be a rocket scientist with a fancy formula, either, although experimentation and finding what works best for you is part of the process. You have to know what you're looking for, so keep your goals in mind here as well.

Reading Your Program Sheets

Every exercise listed on your program sheets will completely work a particular muscle or muscle group. *Blank program sheets, as well as an Exercise Selection Guide to help you in designing a program, are presented later in this chapter.*

While the programs vary, most of the basic exercises stay the same. That way, you can learn and practice good form and technique. These exercises are your nuts and bolts—the chief ingredients, just like in a recipe. Every cake you bake has flour, eggs, liquid, baking powder, and baking soda. The flavor is added with extras: chocolate, nuts, vanilla, cinnamon, etc. You can change the flavor simply by changing your extras. Strength training is similar: Start with basics and add on from there.

Learning your way around the program sheet will help you learn your way around the gym; I've designed it to get you through your workout efficiently. Let's start at the top. Take out the introductory sheet and let's go through it, keeping in mind the same information will apply when you read any of the other programs.

I recommend you train on nonconsecutive days, two or three times a week maximum, then continue with this same number of training sessions each week. You can get excellent results from training just two times a week—if you train with good form and follow all the training tips listed in the captions. However, you'll progress a little quicker if you're training three days per week.

Each sheet has enough space for you to fill in the number of reps, sets, and weight used in your session for three to five weeks. If you increase your workout slowly as I've designed it, each program will take you about eight to ten weeks to complete. So you'll want to photocopy whichever program you're working on so you have enough space to keep accurate records of your progression. Noting what you've accomplished each session will be documented proof that you have gotten stronger. *Yeah!*

We talked about the importance of warm-up in chapter 5. I wanted to make sure you didn't forget about it in your excitement to get started, so your warm-up time and illustrations of stretches are shown on the introductory sheet. You also can use this same stretching program for cooldown. By the time you've finished eight to ten weeks and moved on to the next program, you should know them by heart. If you want more stretching for flexibility than what I've shown here, turn to chapter 9 for my relaxing stretch program; there are twenty great exercises to slow down with.

Now, on to cardiovascular training. Each box gradually increases the amount of time per session you need to be aerobically exercising. It might take you one or two weeks to increase your time, depending on *how often* you're working out. All of my programs progress by number of sessions rather than just weeks. This is in order to increase safely without overdoing it.

On the left side of all of your program sheets is a list of body parts and the corresponding exercises to work each muscle group. These will change slightly for each program as well as the number of sets, reps, rest, and weights. If you're not sure of all the terms we'll be talking about in this chapter, go back and review them in chapter 6.

The exercises are arranged from your largest muscle groups to the smallest, so you'll be starting with leg exercises. This doesn't mean you can't *ever* do your back or chest work first. Just make sure that if you switch the order, you're working larger to smaller groups in succession, rather than jumping around from one muscle group to another. There really is a method here to stimulate the best muscle response.

I've listed some guidelines below to help you determine your starting level as well as how to manipulate the components that intensify your program. These guidelines work for setting up any of these programs:

Choosing Your Program Level

If you have no weight-training experience or very little, I urge you to start with the introductory program. If you have been weight training two to three times a week for at least three months, the intermediate program should be a good challenge for you. Program 3—high-intensity training—is for experienced exercisers who have been strength training a minimum of two to three times a week for at least six months. The key to this program is its intensity, not the amount of weight you're lifting, because you'll be doing one group of supersets after the other without rest. So wait to tackle this one until you've built a solid strength foundation.

Use the circuit program (No. 4) as a restarter, for variety, as a time-saver, or to break a plateau. By the time you have progressed through the first three "readymades," you can design your own. After three or four months, you'll be more familiar with the exercises and which ones your body responds best to so you can fine-tune your own goals.

Program Components

Besides exercise selection, other components interplay as major factors in your program design. As you progress, you probably will be increasing your amount of weight and sets. The number of reps you do is dependent upon the amount of weight you're lifting. As we discussed in chapter 6, you have to know what your strength goals are; if you want to train for strength, use heavier weight and fewer repetitions. If you want to train for endurance, use lighter weight and more reps. Again, the target number of reps for any of the programs is eight to fifteen. You should be able to complete each rep with good form, but remember, the last two reps should be challenging. If you can't even do eight reps, adjust your weight because it's too heavy. On the other hand, if you breeze through fifteen reps, the weight is too light.

There are a couple of gray areas around this repetition recommendation for groups such as legs, biceps, and shoulders. The shoulders—your deltoids—comprise a muscle group which seems to respond better to a high volume of work with lighter weights. They're a *small* muscle group, so it's usually a disadvantage to try and work them with heavy weights. Besides, your deltoids work in association with so many of the other exercises. Biceps, on the other hand, respond well to heavier weight training. If you really want to build your biceps, I've found it redundant to use very light weights. When it comes to biceps, I limit the number of reps with my male clients to only six to eight, because the biceps can be a very stubborn muscle to train, and it's overtrained easily.

One more thing about weight: Just because you're using the more advanced programs doesn't mean you have to be doing it with heavier weights. You can assess your body type, then use the weight levels appropriate for what you want to accomplish. The key is changing the program often, every eight to ten weeks, regardless of the amount of weight you lift. It's about your form and skill, about shocking the muscle and staying fresh and avoiding plateaus. By changing your exercises, number of reps and sets, amount of weight and length of rest, you can overload your muscles to keep them surprised, thus constantly changing and responding.

Remember to rest in between sets, exercises, or supersets. You can shorten your rest period if your goal is to improve muscle endurance, but don't skip it; your muscles need time to recover. On the average, take approximately thirty to forty seconds break time, but no more than a minute and a half. This gives your muscles enough downtime to be able to get through another set.

If you're too tired to do another set, examine the amount of rest you're taking and the amount of weight that you're lifting. You need to listen to your body. The intermediate and high-intensity training programs recommend no rest between exercises, but that doesn't mean you can't stop. The idea is to get through *each superset*, stopping only long enough to reset a position for the next exercise. By keeping your rest period at a minimum *between* supersets, you'll be increasing the intensity of the workout.

∾

Ready-Made Programming

The Introductory Program

The introductory program is just that. There are eleven key exercises, one for every major muscle group, plus three "core" exercises that zero in on abdominals. I think of the introductory program as being for any body type and for just building up a basic foundation. You're strengthening all your major muscle groups in order to build a solid foundation. This foundation will support your future structure. This is a thorough, all-around program for anyone to start with.

Look at the introductory program sheet; you'll notice it says to do one set of fifteen reps for day one. On the second day, it says to do one or two sets; but if it's been three or four days since you've been able to get to the gym, do one set again instead of progressing, because you probably won't be ready to move on yet. Also, if completing one set with all the recommended reps was really difficult for you, stick with only one set again as well. You're setting out on a life of fitness, and you don't have to do it all at once. You'll have more chance to stick with it if you start out a little slower and are consistent with it.

Intermediate Program

For the intermediate program, you'll be doing more exercises, but it's not necessarily going to take you more time. In the introductory program, you only did one or two exercises per muscle group. Now you're going to combine exercises into supersets so that you're doing three exercises in a row per muscle group. Instead of resting between your exercises, you're going to be doing *active* rest by working your opposing muscle groups. This means that while one group is resting, another muscle group is working. This is a very time-efficient approach to training and a little bit more intense than repeating the same exercise with a rest between sets, although you'll still do three sets of a superset before going on to the next muscle group.

You'll probably also burn more calories, although aerobics is considered the real calorie-burning exercise. If you're lifting weights and you're not sitting around much with a lot of rest, don't for a minute think that you're not burning calories! But bear in mind that, in order to change a muscle, you need to fatigue it, so doing twenty-five repetitions with five pounds might not be effective—especially if you haven't fatigued the muscle. In this case, you'd definitely need to add some more weight. Besides, doing twenty-five repetitions takes approximately twice the amount of time. I'd rather do it in half the time!

Some of my clients, whose legs respond quickly and tend to build up from using heavy weights, do better with a lighter weight and different exercises than someone with different genetics. With someone like Cher, who has stubbornly thin legs, she needed to use very, very heavy weights with a low-rep range in order to build any shape in her legs. If I followed her program, I would end up looking like a mud wrestler, because my legs tone easily, even with the slightest weight.

With Susan Dey on the other hand, I used completely different methods from Cher. Susan has knee problems, and she cannot tolerate heavy weights because she would experience terrible pain in her joints the next day. She does very, very light, high-volume work, and her legs are very defined, sharp, and hard looking with a lot of separation in her quads. She works around the twenty- to twenty-five-rep range and does a lot of supersets, which works well for her. She is in the intermediate-to-advanced leg-work stage, even though she's using the very light weights.

So you have some freedom here to adapt reps and weight within the supersets. You'll also find you have to adapt the amount of weight that you're lifting to the muscle group you're working. You might be able to incline fly with twenty-five pounds in each hand, but you probably won't be using the same dumbbells for lateral raises in the same superset. *That* would be heavy-duty lifting!

High-Intensity Training

This is one of my favorite methods; I love to train with back-to-back supersets. It's such a challenge! By the time you get to this level, you should be proficient in training technique and be able to setup in proper form for the next exercise with minimal rest. High-intensity training provides maximum, muscular overload with two to three supersets per body part, plus two to three isolation exercises to top it off. This is truly efficient training. If you're seasoned in strength training and *starting* with this program, but more used to single exercise training, you can expect to see significant body-shaping changes from this program. You might often need to lighten the poundage to get through without any rest.

Circuit Training

If you're restarting, even if you had been training at higher intensities previously, this is a good program to come back with. You might even find the amount of weight you can lift now is more than what you could lift when you initially did this program. That's because your muscles *do* have a memory, and it doesn't take much to retrigger them into action.

The circuit program can also be used for variety training at any level, as well as for a specific activity that you continue to use for one to two weeks as a plateau blaster. Circuits are great, too, if one of your primary goals is weight loss, because of the continuous activity of moving from one exercise to another. Also, if you feel stale and uninspired by your current program, a circuit is an energy shot in the arm to stimulate your muscles as well as your motivation.

Most circuits are based on time, rather than weight and reps. This circuit alternates upper and lower body exercises for thirty to forty-five seconds each, thereby creating a built-in rest period, so you don't have to stop. Complete as many reps with as good a form as possible in the amount of time allotted. Once you go through all the exercises in the order shown, repeat it two or three rounds, depending upon your fitness level.

The beauty of circuit training is that you can alternate the resistance exercises with cardiovascular training, for a more endurance-based workout. This can be a real time-saver if you're running late, and don't have time for both an aerobic and strength workout.

For example, do your squats and lat pulldowns for thirty to forty-five seconds each, followed by two to three minutes of step or another form of cardio. After that, move on to the next couple of exercises on the sheet, followed by another cardio session. Continue until you have completed all the exercises on the program sheet.

Notice on the bottom of the Program 4 sheet that I've recommended some additional cardiovascular work; this is optional, depending on how many sets of the circuit you did and if you included any cardio as part of the circuit. Also, once you've cooled down, do your abdominals, back, and stabilization exercises. I feel these exercises really need your mental concentration and should be done separately.

Designing Your Own Program

One of the nice things about all the information I'm giving you is that you'll know your body well enough to be able to structure a program to shape your body in a way that *you* want it to look. That's the power of weight training. You truly can have an amazing amount of control over how you want to shape your muscles.

Use the training tips at the end of every caption in chapter 8 to help you get the "feel" of each exercise. If you're doing a lat pulldown behind the neck, let's say, and you really *feel* that in your lats—you can feel the lats working well and the blood flowing into them—that's probably going to be a very good exercise to keep in your program. However, if the other lat exercises in the program don't give you that same complete feel, try a different variation until you find one that does.

Remember to concentrate on the feeling of the muscle working, actually contracting through the entire exercise. If a rope triceps pushdown gives you a better feel than a bar triceps pushdown, then do the rope pushdown for a while. You can still vary the program.

What I've found to be most effective is to keep one core exercise—the one that works each muscle group that gives you the best feel—and vary the other ones around it. You can change the order or the actual exercise selection, but this way you never miss out on the meat and potatoes.

As you choose the exercises you want for your program, you might want to make some notes to yourself as to which exercises feel particularly good when you're doing them, so that when you actually design your program, you'll already know, for example, "Yes, that French press, it just gets my triceps in the best way for the entire contraction; I feel the stretch; I'm comfortable in the position; I look forward to doing it; it motivates me; it's an exercise I enjoy." Guess what? You'd do well to include it in your program.

When I design programs for clients, I ask them, "What exercises do you get a really good feel from?" I choose the exercise that they get the most from; it's their body telling me something. Listen to your body.

∾

A yawn is a silent shout.
—G.K. Chesterton

∾

Exercise Selection

Let's face it, with certain body types and frames, there are weights you'll *never* be able to lift. If you're an ectomorph, you'll never be doing eighty-five-pound dumbbell curls, no matter how many times you try to progress. Form and safety are the most important aspects of any and every exercise you choose. Mental focus, alignment, and correct technique are the important things, because if you do an exercise incorrectly, at worst you might hurt yourself; at best, you won't get any results at all, which can be very disappointing.

Not every body responds to exercises the same way. Susan Dey, for example, can do walking lunges, but she cannot do a forward lunge because pushing back from the lunge position hurts her. In the walking lunge, she can follow it through without having to stop abruptly. The point is, if she didn't know a variation, she'd think, I can't do lunges, they hurt my knees. Lunges are not for everyone, and that's why I've given you variations to work the same muscle groups. You might be surprised that you can do a particular type of lunge, even if other types don't work for you at all.

If you find a certain exercise is uncomfortable, you might want to check the variations listed for each caption as well as the exercise selection sheet, and see if there's another variation that works the same muscle group and feels better to you. Exercise programs are written on a general level, but must be interpreted on a specific level, depending on your body and how it responds to certain movement. What this does is give you the opportunity to find what movements really work for you. You'll know whether it works for you or not because you'll be able to feel it.

When I do an incline fly, it hurts my shoulder; but I can do an incline press, which still works the upper part of my chest without aggravating my shoulder. It's a variation that works for me. Think about variations as a menu from which you get to choose what entrees—and also the condiments—that best suit your tastes and needs. It's also important that you're honest with your choices and careful that you don't replace an exercise with one for a different muscle group. Each program is designed in a very balanced way, and you want to make sure, if you're replacing an exercise, it's for the *same* body part. Don't be tempted to say, "I don't want to work my outer thighs because it's my inner thighs that I hate." That would be like skipping your main course and having two desserts.

There's no such thing as "spot reduction." You can exercise your inner thighs till "the cows come home," and it's not going to get rid of any of the fat deposited there. Be realistic about it. Sometimes we hate exercises, although they're good for us. So, if you're replacing an exercise, be very honest with yourself about why you're replacing it and what you're replacing it with, and you'll come up with a good, healthy program for yourself. The beauty of training is that if you don't like the results you're getting from an exercise, it's simple: replace it with a different one. No result is permanent.

The exercise selection sheet is a helpful guide to choosing variations. Each exercise identifies what level the exercise is on and what equipment you can use to perform it. You'll notice that some exercises are more adaptable to levels and equipment than others. You'll need to try them and see what feels best to you and what ultimately will give you the results for which you're looking. Remember, there's always another exercise, always another position, always an adaptable way.

Stalemate: When to "Up the Ante"

One of the questions I get asked the most is, "When should I change my program?" The longer you've been training, the more you'll need to change your program. I generally find that if someone comes to me who has been very sedentary, I'll keep them in the same program for six to eight weeks, just to let their bodies habituate. That way, they get a chance to really learn the exercise, to know when to push and when to pull, how to relax the opposing muscle group and stabilize their abdominals, and just learn how to work with their bodies.

When you're learning, it's extremely important *not* to move too quickly. Let your body get familiar enough with the exercises to reach a point where you've stopped making the gains—*then* move on, but always in sensible increments. Don't be in too much of a rush to progress and not take full advantage of each program.

We all build and adapt at different rates. If you've been doing a program for eight weeks, but still don't feel comfortable, confident, or know exactly what muscle you're working or where to push from, stay with it a little longer. It's not going to hurt you to get to know your body more specifically by working with those exercises more.

In general, you should be able to increase the amount of weight at least two or three times in five- to ten-pound increments before you're ready to change your program. After increasing the weight that many times—and if you're working at the maximum reps and sets I've recommended and your body seems to be slowing its response—it might be time to change the program *format.* You might be ready to progress to the next level of training to restimulate your muscles.

Beginning on page 184, you will find the Program Design sheets for your use. Note that each right-hand page is a continuation of the chart shown on the preceding left-hand page. For your convenience, it is suggested that when using the program design chart, you open the book sideways and lay it out flat. Following is a sample for how you fill out each chart as you progress in your program. When it comes to core sets, do the following: for all abdominal exercises, do one set of 10-30 repetitions; for back exercises, begin with one set of 5 repetitions and progress up to one set of 15 repetitions; for stablization exercises, begin with one set of 5 repetitions and progress up to one set of 15 repetitions.

Sample										
Squat	10 / 50	10 / 50	15 / 50	15 / 50	10 / 60	10 / 60	15 / 60	15 / 60	10 / 70	10 / 70

Note: In the bottom space, record the weight used; the upper half can be used to record reps.

EXERCISE SELECTION CHART

Beginner level = B; Intermediate level = I; Advanced level = A

VARIATION	Bar-bell	Dumb-bell	Ma-chine	Body Wgt.	Cable	Power Flex Band	Spri Bar	Ankle Wgt.	Step Trnr.	Band	Incl Flat Decl.
EXERCISE											
Lower Body:											
Squat	IA	IA	BIA	BIA		I	I				
Plie		IA	IA	IA		I	I				
Lunges:											
stat.	IA	IA	IA	BI		I	I		IA		
fwd.	IA	IA		I					IA		
rear		IA	IA	BI		I	I		IA		
walk		IA		BI							
Leg curl			BIA		IA		B			BI	
Leg ext.			BIA	BI			B			BI	
Inner thigh			BIA	BI	IA			IA	BIA		
Outer thigh		IA	BIA	BI	IA	IA		IA	BIA	IA	
Calf raise	IA	IA	BIA	BI		I					

EXERCISE SELECTION CHART

Beginner level = B; Intermediate level = I; Advanced level = A

VARIATION	Bar-bell	Dumb-bell	Ma-chine	Body Wgt.	Cable	Power Flex Band	Spri Bar	Ankle Wgt.	Step Trnr.	Band	Incl Flat Decl.
EXERCISE											
Upper Back:											
Lat pulldown:											
rear			BIA	A	IA		B				
reverse grip			BIA	A	IA		B				
close grip			BIA	A	IA		B				
Row:											
single arm			BIA		IA	B				B	
close grip			IA		IA	BI	BI		B		
wide grip			IA		IA	BI	BI		B		
reverse grip	BIA		BIA	B	IA	I			BI		

Chest:									
Fly		BIA	BIA		IA	I		BI	BIA
Press	BIA	IA	BIA			I		BI	BIA
Cable cross			BIA		IA	I		I	
Push-ups:									
Knees				BI					
Toes				IA					
Shoulders:									
Lateral raise		BIA	BIA	B	A		BI		IA
Military press	BIA	IA	BIA	B		BI	B	BI	BIA
Upright row	BIA	IA	BIA		IA	BI	B		
Triceps:									
French press	IA	A	IA		IA	BI	B	I	IA
Pushdown		BIA	BIA		BIA	BI		I	
Kickback	BIA	BIA			IA		B	BI	
Dips				BIA					

EXERCISE SELECTION CHART

Beginner level = B; Intermediate level = I; Advanced level = A

VARIATION	Bar-bell	Dumb-bell	Ma-chine	Body Wgt.	Cable	Power Flex Band	Spri Bar	Ankle Wgt.	Step Trnr.	Band	Incl Flat Decl.
EXERCISE											
Biceps:											
Curl	BIA	BIA	BIA		IA	BI	BI	B		BI	
pronating		IA			IA	BI		B		BI	
concentration		IA	IA		IA	BI		B		BI	
Preacher	IA		BIA		IA						
Lower back:											
Hyperextension			IA	BIA							
Prone Op. arm/leg lift		IA		BIA				IA	I		
Bridging				BIA				IA			

Abdominals:

Curl	IA	BIA	IA	BIA
Obliques	IA	BIA	IA	BIA
Stabilization		BIA		BIA
Reverse		BIA	IA	BIA

PROGRAM 1: INTRODUCTORY

(Do at least two to three times per week for eight to ten weeks: Photocopy at least ten copies for your future use.)

Date *(Fill in)*

Warm-up *(Minutes)*	5-10	5-10	5-10	5-10	5-10	5-10	5-10	5-10	5-10
Cardiovascular *(Min.—Mod.Pace)*	15	15	15	15-20	15-20	15-20	20	20	20
Resistance Exercises *(Sets)*	1	1-2	2	2	2-3	2-3	3	3	3

Stretches (Warm up and cool down. Hold 30-40 seconds.)

(Rest 30-45 seconds between sets.)

LEGS	Squat
	Leg extension
	Leg curl
BACK	Lat pulldown
	Reverse fly

CHEST & DELTOIDS Incline fly									
Chest press									
Lateral raise									
ARMS Triceps									
Biceps curl									
CORE SETS (ONE SET ONLY) Back extension	5	5	5	5	5	7	7	7	7
Abdominal curl (2 counts)	15	15	15	20	20	20	30	30	30
Oblique twist (Alternate sides)	10	10	10	15	15	15	20	20	20
Reverse curl (2 counts)	10	10	10	15	15	15	20	20	20

PROGRAM 2: INTERMEDIATE

(Do at least two to three times per week for eight to ten weeks: Photocopy at least ten copies for your future use.)

Date *(Fill in)*

Warm-up *(Minutes)*	5-10	5-10	5-10	5-10	5-10	5-10	5-10	5-10	5-10
Cardiovascular *(Min.—Mod.Pace)*	20-25	20-25	20-25	25	25	25	25-30	25-30	30

Stretches *(Warm up and cool down. Hold 30-40 seconds.)*

Resistance Exercises
(2-3 sets for single exercises, 30-40 seconds rest in between; 3 sets with no rest between supersets; 8-15 reps.)

LEGS

- Squat
- Lunge
  (Alternate)
- Calf raise
- Leg extension
  (Alternate)
- Leg curl

LEGS	Inner thigh
	(Alternate)
	Outer thigh
BACK	Rev. grip pulldown
	(Alternate)
	Reverse fly
	D.B. row
CHEST & DELTOIDS	Incline fly
	(Alternate)
	Lateral raise
	Bench press
	(Alternate)
	Upright row

PROGRAM 2: INTERMEDIATE (CONTINUED)

(Do at least two to three times per week for eight to ten weeks: Photocopy at least ten copies for your future use.)

Date *(Fill in)*

Warm-up *(Minutes)*	5-10	5-10	5-10	5-10	5-10	5-10	5-10	5-10	5-10
Cardiovascular *(Min.—Mod.Pace)*	20-25	20-25	20-25	25	25	25-30	25-30	25-30	30

Stretches *(Warm up and cool down. Hold 30-40 seconds.)*

Resistance Exercises
(2-3 sets for single exercises, 30-40 seconds rest in between; 3 sets with no rest between supersets; 8-15 reps.)

BICEPS, DELTS, & THIGHS

- D.B. pronated curl
- *(Alternate)*
- Military press

- Preacher curl
- *(Alternate)*
- French press

- Kickback

CORE SETS (ONE SET ONLY)

	10	10	10	12	12	12	15	15	15	15
Hyperext. hands across chest										
Reverse curl										
Oblique twist (right)										
Reverse curl										
Oblique twist (left)										
Stabilization exercises										

PROGRAM 3: HIGH-INTENSITY TRAINING

(Do at least two to three times per week for eight to ten weeks: Photocopy at least ten copies for your future use.)

Date *(Fill in)*

Warm-up *(Minutes)*

| 5-10 | 5-10 | 5-10 | 5-10 | 5-10 | 5-10 | 5-10 | 5-10 | 5-10 |

Cardiovascular *(Min.—Mod.Pace)*

| 30-35 | 30-35 | 30-35 | 35 | 35 | 35 | 35-40 | 35-40 | 35-40 |

Stretches *(Warm up and cool down. Hold 30-40 seconds.)*

Resistance Exercises
(2-3 sets for single exercises, 30-40 seconds rest in between; 3 sets with no rest between supersets; 8-15 reps.)

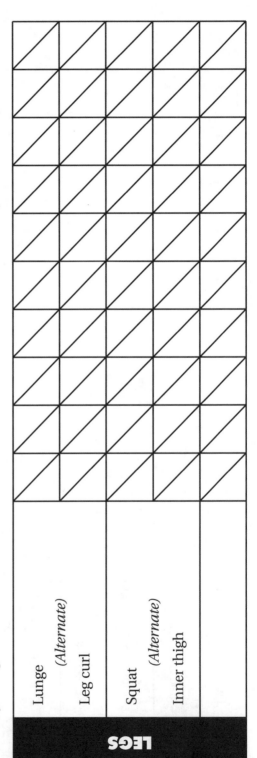

LEGS

- Lunge
  - *(Alternate)*
- Leg curl
- Squat
  - *(Alternate)*
- Inner thigh

LEGS

- Leg extension *(Alternate)*
- Outer thigh
- Calf raise

BACK & DELTS

- D.B. row
- Close-grip pulldown *(Alternate)*
- Reverse fly
- Wide-grip lat pulldown *(Alternate)*
- Straight arm extension

PROGRAM 3: HIGH-INTENSITY TRAINING (CONTINUED)

(Do at least two to three times per week for eight to ten weeks: Photocopy at least ten copies for your future use.)

Date *(Fill in)*

Warm-up *(Minutes)*	5-10	5-10	5-10	5-10	5-10	5-10	5-10	5-10	5-10
Cardiovascular *(Min.—Mod.Pace)*	30-35	30-35	30-35	35	30	35	35-40	35-40	35-40

Stretches *(Warm up and cool down. Hold 30-40 seconds.)*

Resistance Exercises
(2-3 sets for single exercises, 30-40 seconds rest in between; 3 sets with no rest between supersets; 8-15 reps.)

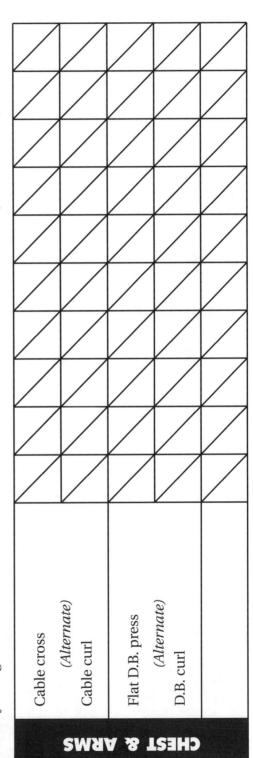

CHEST & ARMS

Cable cross

(Alternate)

Cable curl

Flat D.B. press

(Alternate)

D.B. curl

Incline fly									
(Alternate) Triceps dip									
Cable raise									
Military press									
(Alternate) Upright row									
French press									
(Alternate) Rope pushdown									
Concentration curl									
Lower back and abs									

CHEST & ARMS

DELTS & ARMS

PROGRAM 4: CIRCUIT TRAINING

(Do at least two to three times per week for eight to ten weeks: Photocopy at least ten copies for your future use.)

Date *(Fill in)* _____ _____ _____ _____ _____ _____ _____ _____ _____ _____

Warm-up *(Minutes)* 10 10 10 10 10 10 10 10 10 10

Stretches *(Warm up and cool down. Hold 30-40 seconds.)*

The Circuit
(30-45 seconds for each exercise at a weight which fatigues; no rest between—do cardio between rounds if desired.)

Squat										
Lat pulldown										
Push-up										
Lunge										
Lateral raise										

Triceps dip	D.B. row	Leg extension	Incline fly	Reverse fly (on incline bench)	Leg curl	Biceps curl		

PROGRAM 4: CIRCUIT TRAINING (CONTINUED)

(Do at least two to three times per week for eight to ten weeks: Photocopy at least ten copies for your future use.)

Date *(Fill in)*

Warm-up *(Minutes)* 10 10 10 10 10 10 10 10 10 10

Stretches *(Warm up and cool down. Hold 30-40 seconds.)*

Extra Cardio (5-10 minutes)										
Lower back-Bridging	10	10	10	12	12	12	15	15	15	15
Ab curl	30	30	30	30	30	40	40	40	40	40
Obliques	20	20	20	30	20	30	30	30	30	30
Stabilization	30	30	30	30	30	30	30	30	30	30

Reverse curl	30	30	30	30	30	40	40	40	40	40

PROGRAM 5: SELF-DESIGNED

(Choose evenly between opposing muscle groups.)

Date *(Fill in)* ——— ——— ———

Warm-up *(Minutes)*

Cardiovascular *(15-45 Min.—Mod.Pace)*

Stretches *(Warm up and cool down. Hold 30-40 seconds.)*

Resistance Exercises / Stretches *(Sets)*

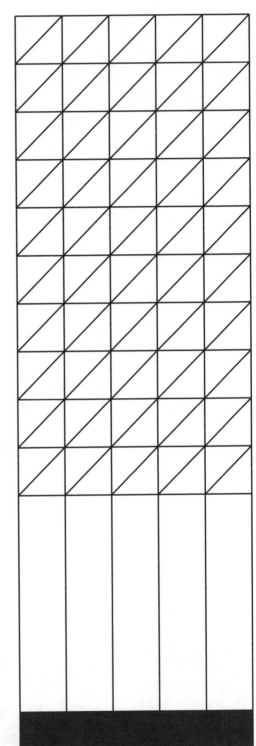

Notes

Notes

Notes

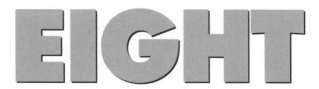

EIGHT

Strength-Training Exercises: *Lower Body*

DISCIPLINE

Without discipline,
there's no life at all.
—Katherine Hepburn

The following exercises, spread out over three chapters, are my favorites to tone and strengthen the muscles "down under." Squats and lunges are like the meat and potatoes of every lower-body training program because the muscles of your thighs and buttocks all work together in a symphony. Depending on the variation, the exercise may use the calves and inner and outer thighs, too.

These exercises develop the greatest amount of shape and tone in the least amount of time, when compared to other exercises. When my clients are running late or short on time, and they still want to do some leg work, I'll sometimes give them just one good, hard set of squats or lunges, and they find they're still getting a great overall lower body workout.

Exercises such as squats and lunges are called multimuscle, multi-joint activities because they use large groups of muscles at the same time. Therefore, they mimic daily activities such as climbing stairs, bending to lift an object, or even getting out of a car. That's why squats and lunges also are ideal for strengthening back muscles and knees, improving overall posture, and making everyday movements easier. You will excel in your life performance. For example, you spend much of your life moving around in an upright mode. By strengthening these same muscles in similar positions that you use in your daily life, these movements naturally become effortless.

Turn to the Exercise Selection Chart in chapter 7 to use as a guideline for developing your own exercise program. The chart cross-references each of the following thirty-eight exercises with recommended equipment variations, and categorizes the programs according to beginner, intermediate, and advanced levels.

SQUAT

(I included regular squatting as part of Cher's program to develop more overall shape and curve to her total lower body and found it to be extremely effective.)

Muscles worked: front of thigh (quadriceps), rear of thigh (hamstring), and buttocks (gluteus maximus)

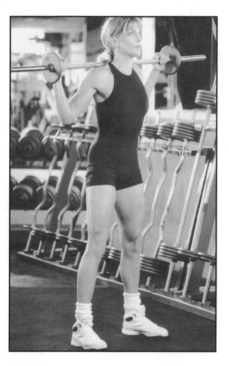 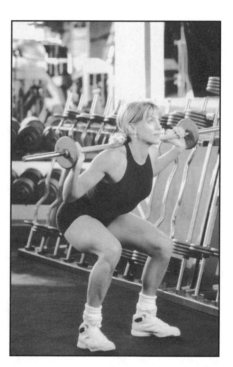

Setup

1. Stand with feet in a comfortable stance about hip-width apart, knees slightly bent, and pelvis in a neutral position with tailbone pointing down.
2. Hold a barbell across the back of your shoulders with an overhand grip a little wider than shoulder-width apart.
3. To keep your torso upright, look straight ahead, squeeze your shoulder blades together, contract abdominals, and lift rib cage.

Action

1. Bend knees and lower your torso toward the floor until hips are even with your knees or just slightly above them.
2. Keep your body weight toward your heels as you squat so your back is straight in a natural extension of the spine, tailbone pointing behind you. Your chin should be tilted slightly upward.
3. Push back up to starting position by straightening your legs in one fluid movement, exhaling as you ascend past the difficult part of the lift.

Training tips

1. Contract abdominals throughout exercise to keep your torso from slouching.
2. Don't lock your knees at any time.
3. As you sit back into the squat, visualize "dunking your tail feathers in a bucket of water behind you."
4. Keep chin lifted; don't look down.
5. Keep heels on the ground so body weight remains to the rear.

Modifications

1. Squat to only a 45-degree angle.
2. For tight calves, use a half-inch plank of wood under the heels to elevate them slightly.
3. Beginners may try a towel squat: wrap a towel around a pole, hold both ends, then squat in the same controlled manner.

Variations

1. Hold a dumbbell in each hand, either on shoulders or by your sides.
2. Narrow stance: Squat with feet only a few inches apart.
3. Toe out to eleven and one o'clock with a slightly wider-than-hip-width stance. This is a great variation if you have tight calves or you want to hit your inner thighs a little harder.

FRONT LUNGE

(We all love to hate lunges; but really we love them, or at least we learn to. The first time I did a set of walking lunges with Cher, she said, "You're a maniac!" But for the next three days, she could barely sit down because of muscle soreness; I made her butt good and sore . . . she was just loving me.)

Muscles worked: front of thigh (quadriceps), rear of thigh (hamstrings), and buttocks (gluteus maximus)

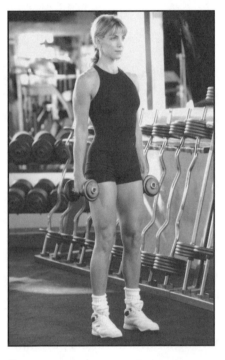 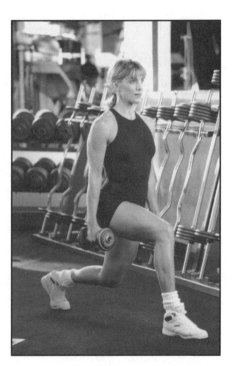

Setup

1. Stand erect in a neutral posture with feet about three to six inches apart and hold a dumbbell in each hand, with palms facing thighs.
2. Contract your abdominals and look straight ahead.

Action

1. Take a large step forward with one foot, leading with the heel, bending both knees so front knee is perpendicular to the floor and in line with ankle, and rear knee points to the floor with heel lifted.

2. Straighten legs and return to starting position by pushing off front heel.
3. Either alternate legs or repeat repetitions with same leg before switching.

Training tips

1. To avoid knee stress, bend front knee only to a 90-degree angle to the ankle (or slightly less).
2. Keep torso erect as you step without leaning forward or backward.
3. Bend knees so front thigh is parallel to the floor.
4. Keep head up and abdominals contracted throughout movement.

Modification

1. If you have knee problems, lunge only to 45 degrees.

Variations

1. Split lunge. Take a large step forward so you're in a wide stride, legs straight but not locked, and back heel up. Bend both knees so front knee is perpendicular to the floor and in line with ankle and rear knee points to the floor with heel lifted. Straighten legs without stepping forward or back and repeat. Keep body weight balanced between front and back legs.
2. Back lunge. Start in the same position. Instead of stepping forward, step backward so knees and torso are in the same alignment as suggested for forward lunge.
3. Walking lunge. Start in the same position. Do a front lunge as described, and bring rear leg forward to meet front foot. Alternate your legs, walking forward in a snipping, decisive movement like opening and closing scissors.
4. Lunge on a step. Do the same lunge, maintaining the same alignment. Rather than step forward on the floor, step forward onto a step six to ten inches high.

INVERTED LEG PRESS

(My client Frank couldn't do squats because of a specific hip problem, but he could successfully leg press without any pain. I find this exercise is a good modification to do instead of squats or lunges if you want one that's easier on the back and knees.)

Muscles worked: front of thigh (quadriceps), rear of thigh (hamstring), and buttocks (gluteus maximus)

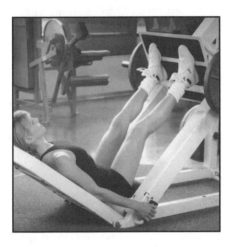
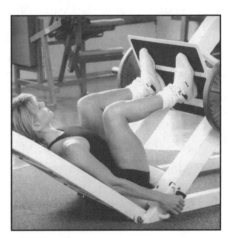

Setup
1. Lie on a leg-press machine with legs extended, knees slightly bent, and feet placed a little wider than hip-width apart in the center of the foot plate.
2. You should have adjusted the backrest so your legs are at a 45-degree angle to your torso.

Action
1. Bend knees in toward chest so knees are just past your hips and you feel a stretch in your buttocks.
2. Straighten legs by pressing out against foot plate until you reach the starting position. Do not lock knees.

Training tips

1. Press firmly and smoothly against the plate as you straighten your legs.
2. Keep back, tailbone, shoulders, and head against rest for the entire exercise.
3. Choose enough weight to challenge the muscles.
4. If you have tight calves, turn feet out to the one o'clock and eleven o'clock positions.

Modifications

1. Bend knees no more than a 90-degree angle.
2. If you have neck discomfort, place a small rolled towel under the neck for support.

Variations

1. Feet together.
2. Feet wider on the plate.
3. Toes turned outward on the plate.

The isolation exercises I've chosen are performed on the leg extension, leg curl, and inner- and outer-thigh machines, and concentrate on working one muscle group and one joint. These exercises are excellent for shaping, gaining strength in a specific area, and joint stabilization.

LEG EXTENSION

(I find the leg extension particularly important for improving the stability of the knee. One of my clients, Marjorie, had chronically sore knees. After we started doing regular leg extensions, she no longer experienced any knee pain.)

Muscles worked: front of thigh (quadriceps)

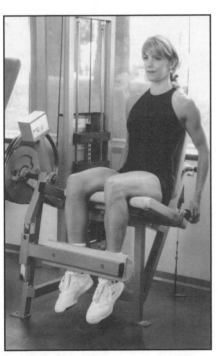
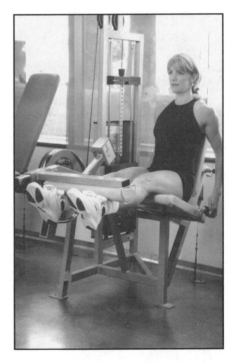

Setup

1. Sit on a leg-extension machine with back pad adjusted at approximately 75 degrees so you're sitting fairly straight with buttocks against the rear of the pad, ankles behind rollers, knees bent, and toes pointed.
2. Grasp handles or edge of seat for support.
3. Contract abdominals and keep torso erect.

Action

1. Straighten legs, pressing against rollers until legs are at hip height, exhaling as you lift.
2. Hold for one to two seconds at top of the lift and slowly return to starting position.

Training tips

1. Don't bounce or jerk the lifting or return motion.
2. Use a weight that allows you to straighten your legs fully through entire range of motion up to hip height without locking knees.
3. Keep toes pointed and rollers adjusted at ankle height, not over toes.

Modification

1. Use an additional seat pad behind your lower back to keep you sitting upright.

Variations

1. Turn toes in or out to stress different parts of the quadriceps.
2. "One-and-a-half": Execute full rep and return only halfway down, return to the top of the movement, and then lower to starting position.

LEG CURL

(The hamstring muscles give the back of your legs the most beautiful shape. One of the best and safest ways of creating this sexy curve is with a correctly performed hamstring curl.)

Muscles worked: rear of thigh (hamstring), some buttocks

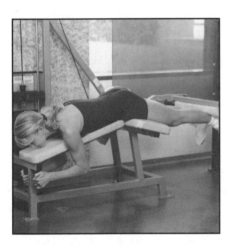 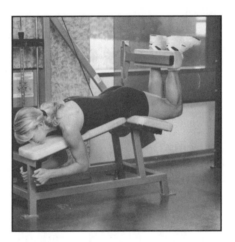

Setup

1. Lie on a leg-curl machine, chin on pad and legs extended so knees are just below edge of the bench and rollers are behind ankles.
2. If it is a flat bench, place a rolled towel underneath the bend at your hips. If the machine has a built-in decline, align the bend in the machine with the natural bend where your hips flex.
3. Tilt pelvis to pull tailbone down toward your feet so your pubic bone is in contact with the bench throughout the movement.

Action

1. Exhale and pull heels up toward buttocks, keeping pubic bone in contact with the pad so you're never arching your back.
2. Keep the feet flexed throughout movement.

3. Hold for one to two seconds at the top of the movement, then slowly return to starting position without hyperextending knees.

Training tips

1. Keep the weight stack slightly suspended throughout movement.
2. Keep head and neck aligned and back straight.

Variations

1. "One-and-a-half": One full rep up, half rep down, half rep up, return to starting position.
2. Turn toes in or out to stress different parts of the hamstring.

OUTER-THIGH MACHINE (Hip Abduction)

(Working your upper hip in this position helps create the "love dent," the great little indentation on the outside of your buttocks.)

Muscles worked: upper hip (gluteus medius)

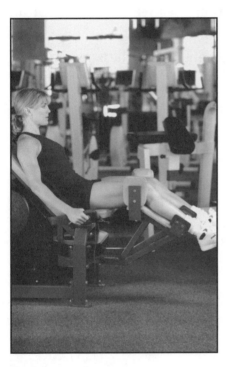 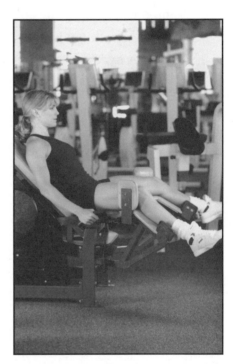

Setup

1. Sit on an abduction machine, holding handles for support with legs extended so leg pads are just above ankle height.
2. Press legs outward against pads so they are hip-width apart. The weight stacks will be slightly lifted.
3. Contract abdominals, keep chest lifted, and look straight ahead.

Action

1. Maintain torso position and press legs outward to about shoulder-width so toes form a diagonal to the shoulder. Hold this position, count "one thousand one," then slowly return to the starting position.

Training tips

1. Contract abdominals firmly throughout movement to keep lower back against pad.
2. Don't separate legs so wide that you can't bring them back together and maintain position.
3. Always use slow, controlled movement.

Modification

1. Use a neck roll if necessary to support cervical spine.

Variation

1. "One-and-a-halves."

INNER-THIGH MACHINE (Hip Adduction)

(While it won't remove excess fat, this exercise offers you a well-toned inner thigh while balancing the strength of the total leg. While there are other ways of working your inner thighs, this machine is very efficient; it creates a great amount of overload in a very short period of time.)

Muscles worked: inner thigh (adductors, pectineus, gracilis)

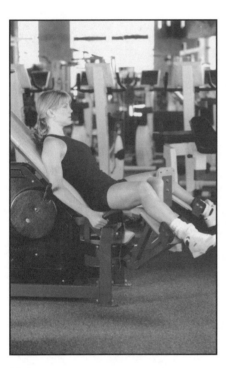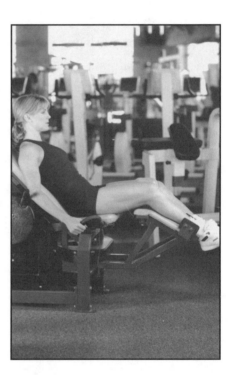

Setup

1. Sit on an adduction machine with back against pad, holding handles for support with legs extended and feet relaxed.
2. Adjust leg pads so that the top pair are just above your knees and the bottom pair are just above your ankles.
3. Separate legs a little farther than shoulder-width so you begin with the inner thighs in a fully stretched position.
4. Contract abdominals to keep lower back in contact with pad; head up.

Action

1. Pull legs together in a very steady, smooth movement until they touch.
2. Resist the machine's outward pull as you open your legs to the starting position so you get the benefit of working in both directions.

Training tips

1. Always start and return to the fully stretched position.
2. Use your abdominals to keep your back against pad.

Modification

1. Use a neck roll to support cervical spine.

Variation

1. "One-and-a-halves."

ONE-LEGGED CALF RAISE

(This is another of Cher's core exercises that we found really effective in giving her calves some shape.)

Muscles worked: calves (gastrocnemius and soleus)

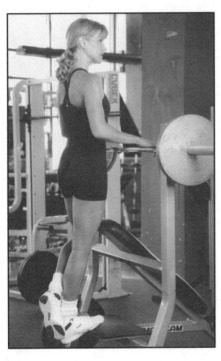 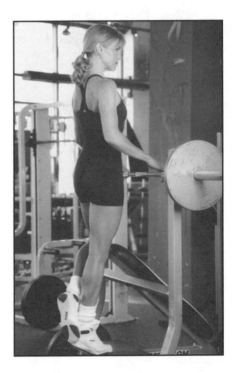

Setup

1. Stand with the ball of one foot on a platform or a bench, and the other foot wrapped around ankle of working leg.

2. Hold on to a support for balance so you can keep torso erect and pelvis in neutral alignment, tailbone pointing down.

3. Drop heel of working leg below the level of the platform until you feel a stretch in your calf.

Action

1. Exhale and slowly elevate up onto the ball of the working foot, keeping torso straight and body weight balanced over ball of foot.
2. Pause at the top of the lift for a count of "one thousand one."
3. Lower to starting position, dropping heel below platform and repeat.

Training tips

1. Avoid rolling body weight out toward little toe; maintain balance over ball of foot.
2. Keep knees relaxed all the way through the movement without locking them.

Variations

1. Hold a dumbbell in the same hand as the working leg.
2. Double calf raise. Drop both heels below the platform and lift up onto balls of both feet at the same time.

Notes

Notes

Notes

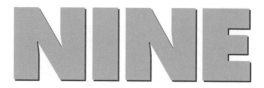
NINE

Strength-Training Exercises:
Upper Body

CONCERN
*should drive us into action
and not depression.*
—*Karen Horney*

'm always amused to find that my female clients believe that training the muscles in their upper body will give them massive muscles (men have more testosterone and can develop larger muscles when training with very heavy weights). What I can assure women of instead is a symmetrical, proportioned torso with well-toned shoulders and arms. Exercises that work your "lats," the largest muscle group in your back, and exercises that develop your shoulders can create the illusion of a "V." So, if you are proportionately larger on the bottom, you can make your waist and hips seem smaller by defining these muscles.

Working your biceps and especially your triceps can give wonderful shape and tone to your arms. Aesthetics aside, don't be deceived and work only the muscles that you can see, such as your chest and arms. Other back exercises, such as the reverse fly, will keep you standing without slouching, and help alleviate back and neck pain that comes from poor posture. Standing straight can often make your body "look" pounds lighter without you even losing an ounce, adding grace and ease to movement. Can you imagine Katherine Hepburn with a slouch?

INCLINE FLY

CHEST EXERCISES: *(I've never been exactly what you call buxom. However, I found that by working my pecs, I developed much more tone, shape, and form to my whole chest area. I like that!!)*

Muscles worked: chest (pectorals), front of shoulder (anterior deltoid), sides of torso (serratus anterior)

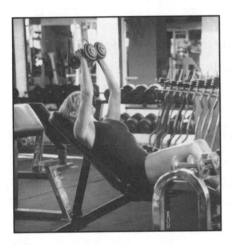
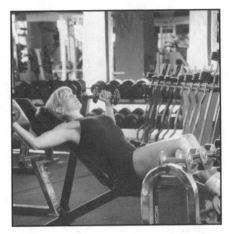

Setup

1. Place the incline bench close to something you can rest your feet on, such as a weight stack, so you can keep your feet up and knees bent with your back against the bench throughout the exercise.
2. Hold a dumbbell in each hand above your collarbone, with palms facing in and wrists straight.
3. Contract abdominals to secure back position against the pad.

Action

1. Bend elbows and lower weights in an arc out to the sides until elbows are in line with your shoulders and you can see weights in your peripheral vision.
2. Slowly press arms up and together, maintaining the same arc, back to starting position.

Training tips

1. Lower weights to the point that you feel a full stretch of the chest muscles; dropping too low can result in loss of control.
2. Don't bounce out of the bottom position; use slow and controlled movement: four counts to lower and two counts to lift.
3. Picture yourself hugging a large tree.

Modifications

1. Use a neck roll to support the cervical spine.
2. Incline cables flies. To further protect your shoulder, set the incline bench between two low cable pulleys and perform the same exercise.

BENCH PRESS

Muscles worked: chest (pectorals), front of shoulder (anterior deltoid), sides of torso (serratus anterior), rear of arm (triceps)

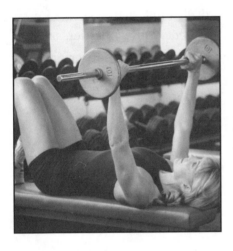 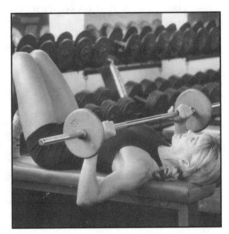

Setup

1. Lie on a weight bench with knees bent and heels on the bench edge, abdominals contracted and back in contact with the bench.
2. Hold a bar with an overhand grip above midchest, a little wider than shoulder-width apart, keeping wrists straight.

Action

1. Stabilize torso by squeezing shoulder blades toward the bench, keeping rib cage lifted.
2. Inhale and bend elbows to lower bar until it is about one inch above the chest.
3. Exhale and slowly push bar back up to starting position without locking the elbows.

Training tips

1. Keep spine in a neutral position so that it doesn't arch during either the lifting or lowering phase of the exercise.
2. Work through a full range of motion, using chest muscles to initiate the movement.

Modification

1. Use a neck roll to support cervical spine.

Variations

1. "One-and-a-halves."
2. Dumbbell press. This is performed the same, but with dumbbells instead of a barbell.

STANDING CABLE CROSS

Muscles worked: chest (pectorals), front of shoulder (anterior deltoid), sides of torso (serratus anterior)

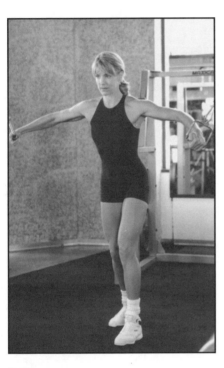 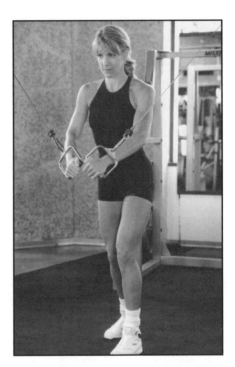

Setup

1. Stand in the center of a high cable pulley machine in a staggered stance with feet hip-width apart and one foot in front of the other.
2. Bend knees slightly and lean torso forward, keeping back straight at an angle of about 10 to 15 degrees.
3. Hold handles with elbows slightly bent just lower than shoulder-height so palms face down and wrists are straight.
4. Squeeze shoulder blades together to lift chest and rib cage; keep abdominals contracted.

Action

1. Exhale and draw arms together until knuckles meet in front of your navel; contract the chest throughout the entire movement.
2. Inhale and release arms in a slow movement, resisting the pull of the cables back to starting position.

Training tips

1. Maintain the same bend at the elbows through the entire range of motion.
2. Make sure you're in a comfortable and supported stance so as you press arms together, your body position doesn't waver to lean farther forward.
3. Use abdominals to keep torso from slouching as arms press together.
4. As you become fatigued, allow a greater bend in the elbows to get some assistance from your triceps.

Modification

1. If you have shoulder problems, turn palms up as arms come together.

PUSH-UP

Muscles worked: chest (pectorals), front of shoulder (anterior deltoid), sides of torso (serratus anterior), rear of upper arm (triceps)

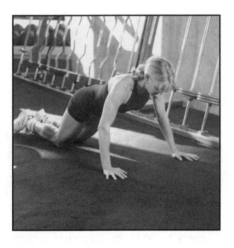 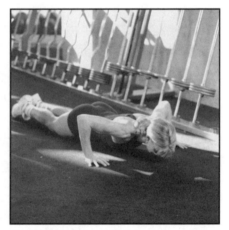

Setup

1. Kneel on all fours; knees are slightly apart and behind hips. Hands are on floor with fingers pointing forward, just in front of shoulder joint, with arms extended a little wider than shoulder-width apart.
2. Contract abdominals and buttocks so your back is straight and in one line from the top of your head to your tailbone.
3. Look about six inches in front of your hands to keep head from dropping.

Action

1. Inhale and lower chest toward the floor, maintaining body position so back doesn't arch or abdominals sag.
2. In the finished position, your chest should be one-half to one inch from the floor with elbows above torso level.
3. Exhale and push back up to starting position without locking elbows.

Training tips

1. Lower and lift body as one movement so head, neck, and back stay aligned.
2. Only lower as far as you can while maintaining alignment and still pushing back up smoothly.
3. Contract abdominals throughout movement.

Modification

1. If you have shoulder or wrist problems, try doing the push-up in a standing position, two to three feet away from a wall with your hands on the wall at shoulder height.

Variation

1. Full push-up. This is performed the same, but with legs extended and ankles crossed. It's more difficult because you're lifting more body weight.

BEHIND-THE-NECK PULLDOWN

BACK EXERCISES: *(While working with me, Susan Dey developed a beautifully flared back. She feels proud of her back, too, and oftentimes wears backless dresses to show it off. We achieved this by doing a mixture of all the following exercises.)*

Muscles worked: middle back (latissimus dorsi, teres major), rear shoulder (posterior deltoid), front of upper arm (biceps)

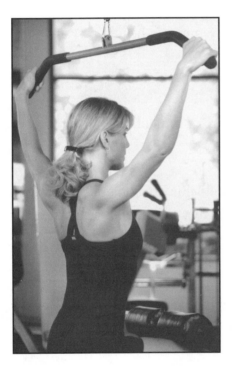 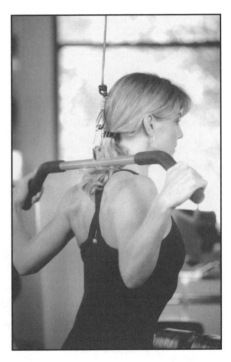

Setup

1. Sit erect on a lat-pulldown machine with thighs under rollers, knees bent, and feet flat on floor.
2. Hold the bar with a wide overhand grip so hands are more than shoulder-width apart, and wrists are straight.
3. Lean forward slightly, about 5 to 10 degrees so that you feel a stretch in the lat muscles.

Action

1. Still holding the bar, inhale and depress the shoulder blades downward and inward as if the lower tips will touch.
2. Follow this movement by exhaling and bending elbows to pull down bar to the base of your neck.
3. Maintain torso position; do not rock forward, but keep spine straight and abdominals contracted.
4. Slowly release bar back to starting position until you feel a stretch in your lats.

Training tips

1. Always start the movement by dropping your shoulder blades first, so that you really get the feeling of using your lats and not just your biceps.
2. Keep head up as you pull bar behind you.

Modification

1. If you are particularly tight in the shoulders and chest region, a narrow-grip pulldown may be a more appropriate choice.

Variation

1. Do the same exercise, but use a different bar or a wider or narrower grip.

REVERSE-GRIP PULLDOWN

Muscles worked: middle back (latissimus dorsi, teres major), upper back (trapezius and rhomboids), shoulders (deltoids), front of upper arm (biceps)

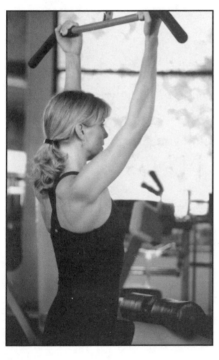 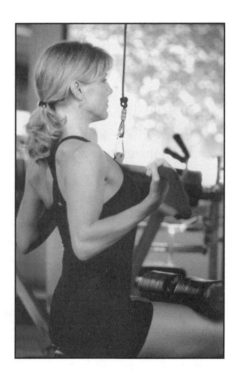

Setup

1. Sit on a lat-pulldown machine with thighs under rollers, knees bent, and feet flat on floor.
2. Hold a bar with an underhand grip about shoulder-width apart, and arms extended so you feel a stretch between shoulder blades as if lat muscles were flared.
3. Keep spine straight, but lean back just slightly as you hold the bar; keep abdominals contracted.

Action

1. Pull shoulder blades down and back before moving arms, then exhale and slowly pull bar down toward upper chest, bending elbows behind you.
2. At the finish of the movement, keep your torso at the same angle without leaning back any farther, while keeping chest open and shoulder blades together.
3. Inhale and slowly return bar to starting position.

Training tips

1. As you pull bar toward chest, it should feel like you're pulling yourself up, rather than pulling bar down.
2. Don't lean back too far; you shouldn't feel strain in your lower back.

Variation

1. Narrow-grip pulldown. The starting position is the same, but you use a short handle so palms are together and facing in. Pull down arms toward upper chest, keeping elbows close to your sides.

STRAIGHT ARM EXTENSION

Muscles worked: middle back (latissimus dorsi, teres major), upper back (trapezius), middle shoulder (lateral deltoid), rear of upper arm (triceps)

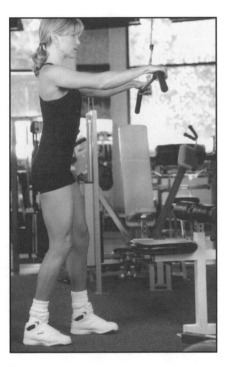 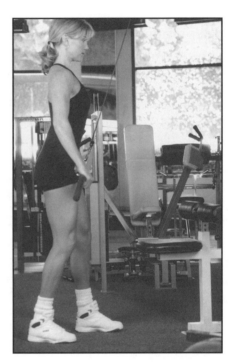

Setup

1. Stand about a foot away from a high cable pulley machine in a staggered stance so that you can hold bar at arm's-length away.
2. Hold bar in an overhand grip at forehead level with hands about shoulder-width apart and wrists straight.
3. Knees and elbows are slightly bent, and shoulders are down and back, with your spine in a neutral position and abdominals contracted.

Action

1. Squeeze shoulder blades down and back, then pull bar down toward thighs, maintaining the same arm and torso position.
2. Slowly return bar to starting position and repeat.

Training tips

1. Only the arms move; keep the rest of the body still as you press down.
2. Keep head up.
3. The arms maintain a constant position, with elbows slightly bent; the arms don't bend or straighten during this exercise.
4. This exercise is excellent when supersetted with a behind-the-neck pulldown or reverse pulldown.

Variation

1. Do the same exercise from a triceps high pulley cable machine, using either the E-Z bar or the rope.

ONE-ARMED DUMBBELL ROW

Muscles worked: middle back (latissimus dorsi, teres major), rear shoulder (posterior deltoid)

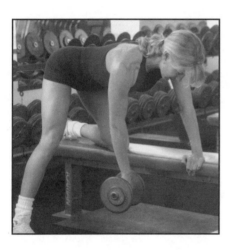 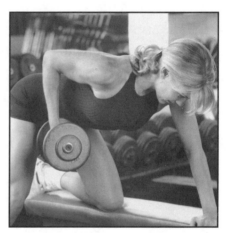

Setup

1. Kneel with left knee on a bench and the right foot flat on floor, knee bent so hips and shoulders are square and back is straight, abdominals contracted.
2. Place left hand about six to eight inches in front of your torso on the right side of the bench, palm turned and arm straight, but not locked.
3. Hold a dumbbell in your right hand, palm facing rear with arms hanging in a straight line from your shoulder, so you feel a stretch around your shoulder blade.
4. Look down at bench so head and neck are aligned with spine.

Action

1. Slowly draw elbow up and slightly above rib cage as you rotate shoulder so palm faces in at the top of the lift.
2. Feel shoulder blades pulling together as you lift.
3. Slowly return to starting position, rotating shoulder so palm faces the rear.

Training tips

1. Lift dumbbell only to waist height, so upper arm is parallel to floor with shoulders square.
2. Don't rotate torso as you lift; the movement is straight up and back.

Variation

1. Do this same exercise using a low cable pulley.

REVERSE FLY

UPPER BACK AND SHOULDERS: (*I love to work the shoulders! They're one of the most attractive muscles in the upper body [and one of the most stubborn to change]. The delts offer a beautiful line to the overall shape of your body when well developed. Kirstie Alley was a swimmer and had a naturally fabulous set of shoulders; she never had to work them hard. Other clients have not been so genetically gifted and have found it has*

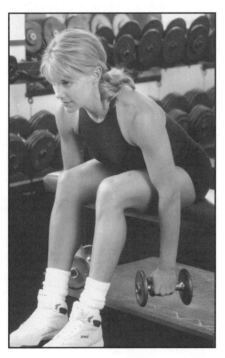 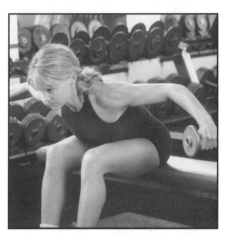

only been through persistent, hard, regular shoulder work that they've had success.)

Muscles worked: upper back (trapezius, rhomboids), middle and rear shoulder (medial and posterior deltoids)

Setup

1. Sit on edge of a bench with knees bent and feet flat on the floor; place a dumbbell behind each heel.
2. Lean forward from your hips so that chest can rest on your thighs; keep back and neck straight so you're not looking up or dropping the chin down.
3. Grasp a dumbbell in each hand, with palms facing in so that your arms hang in line with your shoulders; elbows are slightly bent.

Action

1. Lift arms up and draw shoulder blades together until arms are at shoulder height, with wrists straight and palms down.
2. Keep elbows slightly bent throughout movement, lifting up and away from the body in an arc.
3. Chest stays in contact with thighs so back and neck remain straight.
4. Hold and count "one thousand one" at top of lift, then slowly return to starting position.

Training tips

1. This movement is executed much better with a light weight. It's challenging enough just to maintain the position and lift through the full range of motion.
2. Lead the movement back and up with your elbows, not your hands.
3. Don't jerk torso upward as you squeeze shoulder blades together; maintain body alignment.

Variation

1. If you're uncomfortable in the bent-over position, lie face down on an incline bench, so that your body is elongated.

ALTERNATING DUMBBELL MILITARY PRESS

Muscles worked: upper back (trapezius, rhomboids), shoulders (deltoids), front of upper arms (biceps)

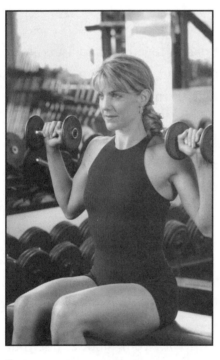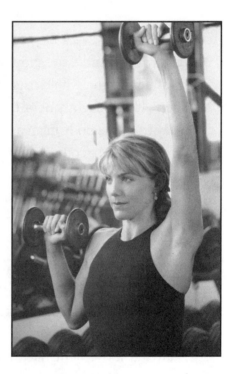

Setup

1. Sit erect on the edge of a bench, knees bent, and feet flat on floor with abdominals contracted and rib cage lifted.
2. Hold a dumbbell in each hand with an overhand grip, elbows bent and close to your sides so dumbbells are positioned in front of your shoulder joint.

Action

1. Straighten one arm without locking elbow, keeping it in line with shoulder, wrist neutral.
2. Squeeze shoulder blades together and hold abdominals tight to keep torso from swaying.
3. Return to starting position and alternate with other arm.

Training tips

1. Raise arm in one fluid motion, without letting arm drift out to the side.
2. Return to starting position before straightening other arm.
3. Use abdominals to keep you sitting upright.

Modification

1. Use a bench that has a backrest to give you more support.

Variations

1. Raise both arms at same time.
2. Do this same exercise standing, which requires more torso stabilization and is more difficult.
3. Use a barbell instead of dumbbells.

UPRIGHT ROW

Muscles worked: upper back (trapezius, rhomboids), front and middle shoulder (anterior and medial deltoid), front of upper arms (biceps)

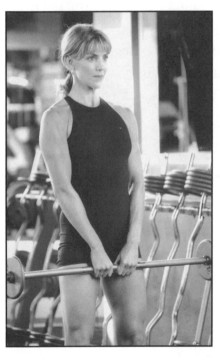 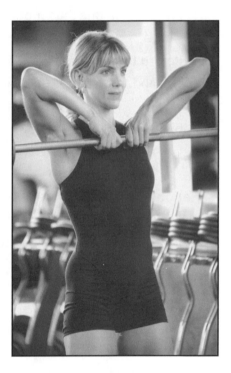

Setup

1. Stand with feet hip-width apart, knees bent, and pelvis in neutral alignment so tailbone points down with abdominals contracted.

2. Hold a barbell in front of thighs with a narrow overhand grip, hands about three inches apart.

Action

1. Maintain torso position, exhale and bend elbows to lift barbell up to collarbone level.
2. In the finished position, elbows will be above shoulder height, with wrists straight.
3. Inhale and slowly lower bar back to starting position, without locking elbows.

Training tips

1. Don't rock torso backward to assist lifting bar.
2. Keep body weight balanced over arches for a firm, neutral base of support.
3. Use abdominals to keep torso upright.
4. This is a great exercise to superset with other upper-body exercises, such as another shoulder exercise, military press, or biceps curls.

Modification

1. If you have shoulder problems, using dumbbells instead of a barbell allows for a greater freedom in range of motion so you can squeeze your shoulder blades together and stabilize easier.

Variations

1. Do this same exercise using a low cable pulley.
2. Use a wide grip so hands are in front of thighs to induce more shoulder work.

LATERAL RAISE

Muscles worked: middle shoulder (medial deltoid)

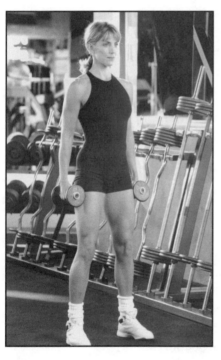 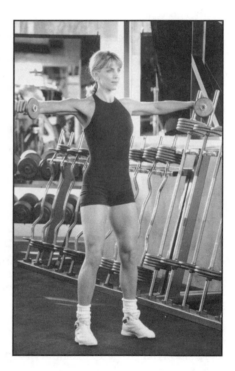

Setup

1. Stand with feet hip-width apart or a little wider, knees bent, and pelvis in neutral alignment, with chest lifted and abdominals contracted.

2. Hold a dumbbell in each hand close to your thighs, palms facing in with elbows slightly bent.

3. Press shoulders back and down, and keep head in line with your spine so your chin doesn't jut forward as you lift.

Action

1. Keep elbows slightly bent, lift arms up and out to the side in four counts until elbows are at shoulder height with palms down.
2. Hold at the top of the lift for a moment, counting "one thousand one," and then lower to starting position in four counts.

Training tips

1. Keep chest lifted; it's a common mistake to try lifting using the trapezius in the upper back instead of the deltoids.
2. Never lift your hands higher than your shoulders (this is a very controlled, precise movement).

Modification

1. If you have neck problems, sit on an incline bench at about 45 degrees, with a towel rolled behind neck. Do the same exercise, lifting hands only up to shoulder height.

SIDE CABLE RAISE

Muscles used: middle and rear shoulder (medial and posterior deltoid)

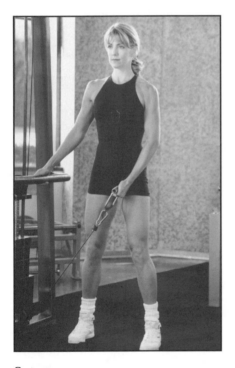 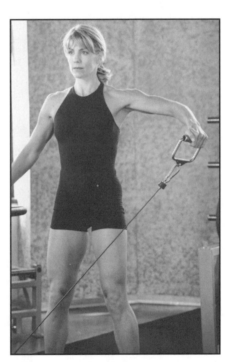

Setup

1. Stand sideways to a low cable pulley machine with feet hip-width apart, knees slightly bent, and pelvis in neutral alignment; keep free hand on hip for support.

2. Grasp the handle in your outside hand with an underhand grip and step away from machine, if necessary, to place slight tension on the cable; the arm is relaxed in front of your thighs, and elbow is slightly bent.

Action

1. Lift arm up and away from torso up to shoulder height in four counts with palm facing down; elbow stays slightly bent through full range of motion.
2. Hold at the top of the lift, counting "one thousand one," then slowly lower to starting position.

Training tips

1. This exercise is a little more advanced than lateral raises because it fully isolates the shoulder muscles, especially the lateral head of the deltoids.
2. Don't jerk the cable as you start to lift upward; this can stress rotator muscles in the shoulder.
3. Contract abdominals firmly to maintain an erect torso.

Modification

1. Lie on your side on an incline bench and lift a dumbbell from your thigh up to shoulder level.

TRICEPS PUSHDOWN

TRICEPS: *(I had a famous client nickname these her "kimono" exercises. I had another call these her "dolman sleeve" exercises. Regardless of what they're called, the strengthened triceps gives your arm the most spectacular, sexy curve. I know that doing these are worth the effort—discomfort, ouch!—when you see the results.)*

Muscles worked: rear of upper arm (triceps)

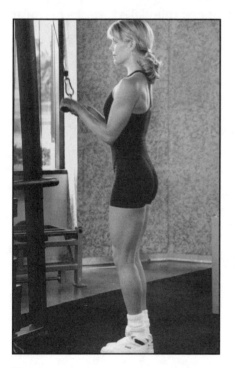 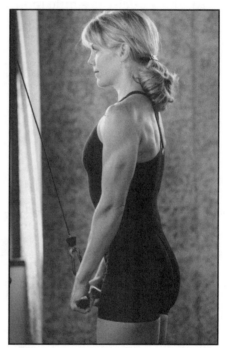

Setup

1. Stand facing a high cable pulley machine with a straight bar attachment, your feet a few inches apart with knees bent, pelvis in neutral alignment, and abdominals contracted.
2. Grasp the bar using an overhand grip with your thumbs on top of the bar. Hold the bar at chest height with elbows bent and pressed close to the front of your waist.

Action

1. Exhale and extend the arms fully without locking elbows until the bar touches the front of your thighs.
2. Keep elbows tucked close to body without flaring outward as you straighten your arms.
3. Maintain neutral, straight wrists throughout movement.
4. Return to starting position using controlled movement.

Training tips

1. Press downward through the hands while keeping elbows in the same position. This forces the triceps to work.
2. Keep head up and back straight so you don't rock back and forth.
3. Keep elbows toward the front of your torso; don't let them drift behind you.

Modification

1. To stabilize the torso, do this same exercise kneeling.

Variations

1. Do the same exercise, using different bars.
2. To superset, do this same exercise, starting with an underhand grip; finish with an overhand grip until fatigued.
3. "One-and-a-halves."
4. Hold a single handle and use one arm at a time to do the same exercise.

ROPE PRESSDOWN

Muscles worked: rear of upper arm (triceps)

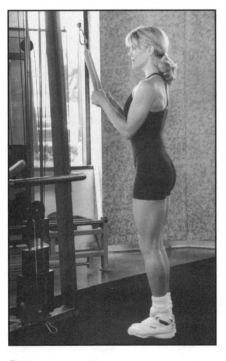
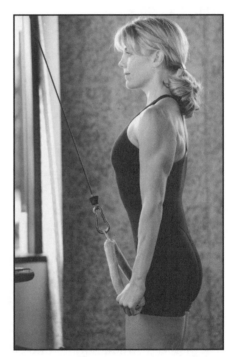

Setup

1. Stand facing a high cable pulley machine with a rope attachment, your feet a few inches apart with knees bent, pelvis in neutral alignment, and abdominals contracted.

2. Grasp the rope above the wooden balls, with palms facing in. Hold the rope at chest height with elbows bent and pressed close to the front of your waist.

Action

1. Exhale and extend the arms fully without locking elbows, separating hands, and turning palms toward the rear at the very end of the movement.
2. Keep elbows tucked close to body without flaring outward as you straighten your arms.
3. Maintain a neutral, straight wrist throughout movement, especially as you rotate palms to the rear.
4. Return to starting position using controlled movement.

Training tips

1. Turn palms toward rear as your arms reach the fully straightened position.
2. Keep head up and rib cage lifted; don't pull torso downward as you pull on the rope.
3. This exercise is best done with light weight.

TRICEPS KICKBACK

Muscles used: rear of upper arm (triceps), rear shoulder (posterior deltoid)

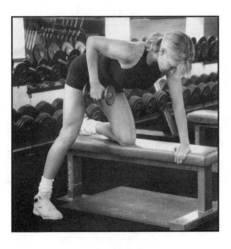 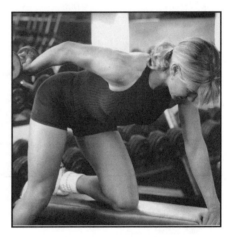

Setup

1. Kneel with left knee on a bench and the right foot flat on floor, knee bent so hips and shoulders are square and back is straight, with abdominals contracted.
2. Place left hand about six to eight inches in front of your torso on the right side of the bench, arm straight but not locked.
3. Look down at the bench so head and neck are aligned with spine.
4. Hold a dumbbell in your right hand, palm in; draw elbow up and slightly above rib cage so dumbbell is at your waist and forearm is perpendicular to the floor.

Action

1. Maintain elbow and shoulder position and extend arm behind you, rotating wrist so palm faces the ceiling at the end of the movement.
2. Hold at the top of the lift, counting "one thousand one," then slowly bend elbow to return to starting position.

Training tips

1. Maintain elbow position a few inches above rib cage throughout the entire exercise; don't let elbow drop as you get tired.
2. Keep head, neck, and spine aligned.
3. Don't rotate torso or shoulders trying to lift arm higher; keep hips and shoulders square.

Variations

1. Do the same exercise, using a low cable pulley.
2. When extending your arm behind you, don't rotate forearm; just bring arm directly behind you.
3. Lie face down on an incline bench; kick back with both arms at the same time.

BARBELL FRENCH PRESS

Muscles worked: rear of upper arm (triceps)

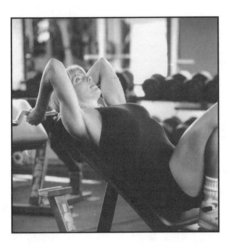 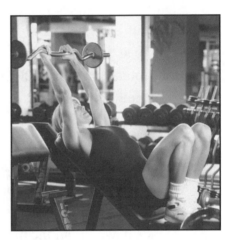

Setup

1. Sit on an incline bench and push your body upward so your buttocks are about six inches off the seat, and knees are bent with heels on the seat's edge. Your head, neck, and back will all be in contact with the rear pad.

2. Hold an E-Z bar in an overhand grip in front of your chest with hands about three to four inches apart.

3. Lift the bar overhead with elbows bent and parallel to each other until bar is slightly behind head and you feel a stretch in your triceps.

4. Keep elbows from flaring by holding them firmly in place in front of you, close to ears.

Action

1. Without changing elbow or shoulder position, straighten arms without locking elbows until bar is above forehead.
2. Pause at the top of the movement, counting "one thousand one," and return to starting position, pausing for the same count of "one thousand one" before lifting again.

Training tips

1. Keep back and head against pad the entire time.
2. Hold the bar behind your head comfortably; don't overstretch so that you can't straighten arms.
3. Superset this exercise with close-grip bench presses of the same weight for added training benefits.

Modifications

1. Do same exercise on a flat bench.
2. For neck problems, use a neck roll.

Variations

1. Do same exercise using a single dumbbell held in both hands.
2. Do with a low or high cable pulley, with your back to the machine.

TRICEPS DIP

Muscles used: rear of upper arm (triceps), shoulders (deltoids)

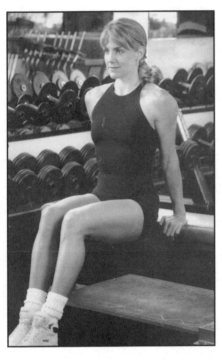 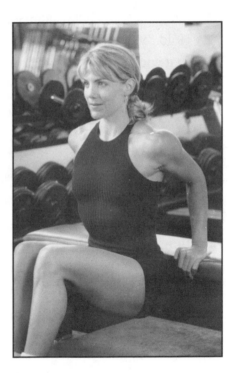

Setup

1. Turn backward to a bench, place hands a little wider than shoulder-width apart on the edge of the bench, arms extended and palms down.
2. Extend legs in front of you so knees are bent at a 90-degree angle, with feet flat on the floor; buttocks should be very close to the bench.
3. Your back should be straight, with abdominals contracted.

Action

1. Bend elbows to lower torso toward the floor, until elbows and shoulders are even, forming almost a 90-degree angle.
2. Keep elbows as close to body as possible, without letting them flare as if they were parallel like railroad tracks.
3. Exhale and push up to starting position without locking elbows, using slow, controlled movement.

Training tips

1. Don't bounce at the bottom of the movement.
2. Keep buttocks close to bench as you lift and lower torso.
3. Keep head up and torso straight.

Modification

1. If you have shoulder or wrist problems and this exercise aggravates these joints, choose an alternate triceps exercise.

Variations

1. Place your feet up on a bench in front of your body, with legs straight and knees soft.
2. Upright dips on a bar or triceps machine that simulates the same action.

BARBELL CURL

BICEPS: *(You'll probably never look like Arnold Schwarzenegger, but flexing a well-toned biceps at a party is a great way to perhaps meet an athletic, potential significant other. On a more serious note, a nicely developed biceps gives great symmetry and balance to your upper arms.)*

Muscles worked: front of upper arm (biceps, brachialis), forearm (brachioradialis)

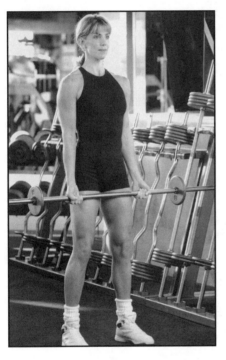 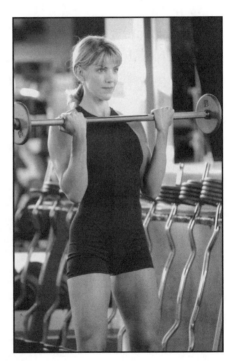

Setup

1. Stand with feet hip-width apart, knees slightly bent, and pelvis in neutral alignment.
2. Hold a barbell with an underhand grip, elbows close to the front of your waist so hands are at the outside of your thighs.

Action

1. Bring barbell up toward chest, while keeping elbows close to your sides.
2. Without locking elbows, return to starting position.

Training tips

1. Keep wrists in neutral position and elbows close to waist.
2. Don't lean backward as you bring the bar toward your chest.

Modification

1. If you have difficulty maintaining alignment in a standing position, do seated dumbbell curls (next page) instead.

Variation

1. Use an E-Z curl bar instead of a straight bar.

SEATED DUMBBELL CURL

Muscles worked: front of upper arm (biceps, brachialis), forearm (brachioradialis)

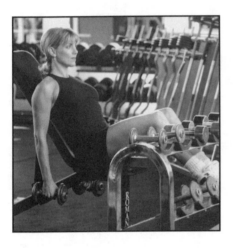 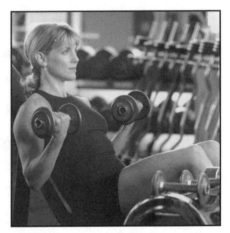

Setup

1. Place an incline bench close to something you can rest your feet on, such as a weight stack, so you can keep your feet up and knees bent with back against the bench throughout the exercise. Incline the bench only slightly at about 45 degrees.
2. Hold a dumbbell in each hand, palms facing in, with arms hanging down in line with your shoulders.

Action

1. Curl dumbbells toward shoulders, elbows close to body, while rotating hands forward through range of motion so palms face torso at the end of movement.
2. Slowly straighten arms and return to starting position.

Training tips

1. Keep elbows pointing down and rib cage lifted with back against pad at all times.
2. Don't swing arms up, but contract biceps to lift arms.

Variations

1. Alternate curls rather than lifting both arms together.
2. Vary the degree of bench incline.
3. Do the same exercise standing.

PREACHER CURL

Muscles worked: front of upper arm (biceps, brachialis), forearm (brachioradialis)

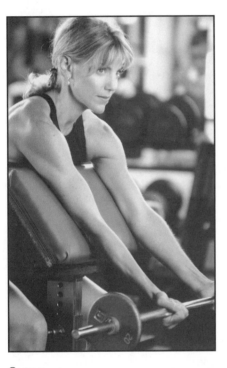 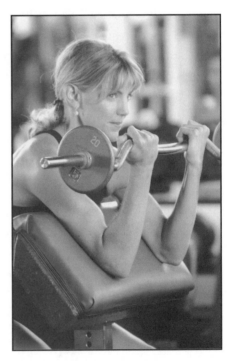

Setup

1. Sit on a preacher curl machine; lean forward so you can hold an E-Z curl bar comfortably, with upper arms and chest resting on support pads.
2. Knees are bent and feet are flat on floor, spine is straight, and abdominals are contracted.

Action

1. Bend elbows and bring bar toward shoulders.
2. Straighten arms to starting position.

Training tips

1. Keep upper arms and chest against pads as you lift.
2. Don't jerk the bar upward; if you have to, this indicates the weight is too heavy; use smooth, controlled movement.

Variations

1. Place a seated preacher curl bench in front of a low cable pulley machine and do the same exercise.
2. Use a preacher curl machine instead of a bench and bar.

STANDING CABLE CURL

Muscles worked: front of upper arm (biceps, brachialis), forearm (brachioradialis)

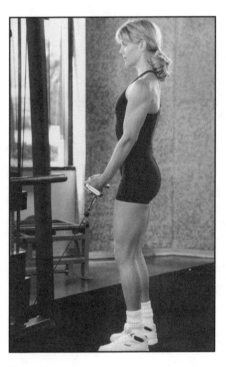
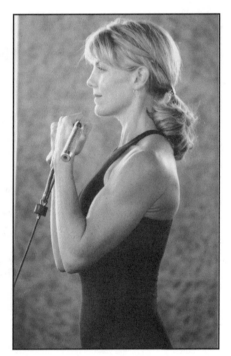

Setup

1. Stand facing a low cable pulley with feet hip-width apart, knees bent, and pelvis in a neutral position.

2. Hold a bar with an underhand grip in front of your thighs, elbows slightly bent; adjust distance from machine so there is some tension on the cable.

3. Keep torso erect without leaning forward or backward, and elbows close to the front of your waist.

Action

1. Without changing elbows or shoulder position, curl bar up toward chest.
2. Return to starting position without locking elbows.

Training tips

1. Don't lean or sway with the body as you lift; keep torso absolutely still.
2. Keep elbows close to your sides for a better biceps contraction as you work through a full range of motion.

Variation

1. Do the same exercise, using one arm at a time, holding a single handle.

CONCENTRATION CURL

Muscles worked: front of upper arm (biceps, brachialis), forearm (brachioradialis)

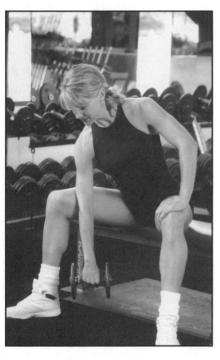 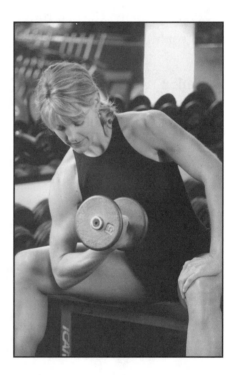

Setup

1. Sit on the edge of a bench with legs separated so you can rest the upper part of your working arm against the inside of your thigh.
2. Hold a dumbbell in your working hand, palm facing rear, wrist straight.
3. Lean slightly forward, keeping back straight; put other hand on thigh for support.

Action

1. Begin to curl dumbbell toward shoulder while keeping a neutral wrist. Rotate arm up and forward through entire range of motion so palm faces shoulder at the top of the lift.
2. Maintain position of the upper arm as a brace while you lift.
3. Slowly straighten arm back to starting position, turning palm to the rear at the bottom of the movement.

Training tips

1. The only movement should be from elbow to dumbbell; the rest of the body and arm are motionless.
2. Use slow, controlled movement; don't jerk the dumbbell toward the shoulder at the top of the lift.

Variations

1. Do the same exercise, using a low cable pulley machine.
2. Stand behind an incline bench with armpits resting on the top of the bench.

Notes

Notes

Notes

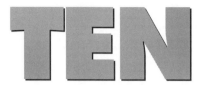

Strength-Training Exercises: *Middle Body*

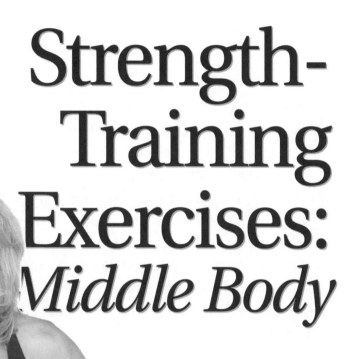

ONE
*can never consent to
creep when one feels the
impulse to soar.*
—Helen Keller

call these "core exercises," and for a good reason. The muscles that make up the midsection, the abdominals, and lower back, along with other major muscles that attach to the pelvis, all work together to stabilize the spine and maintain good posture and alignment when we stand, sit, perform daily activities, and participate in sports.

Our bodies are meant to move, twist, and bend, but when these muscles are out of balance and not strong, injury might occur. As much as you might hate doing them (I do), don't skip these. Core exercises should always be included as part of your weekly routine. People ask me all the time, "How do I get rid of this?" while pointing to their midsection spare tire.

The bottom line is, spot reduction is a myth. It does not exist. Regular cardiovascular work plus a controlled caloric intake will reduce the amount of body fat which might sit on top of the muscle. The combination of losing body fat and doing these exercises make baring your midriff something to be proud of.

ABDOMINAL EXERCISES

Cher was the original abdominizer. She just loved to work her abs, the more the better as far as she was concerned. She was very surprised to see how intense and effective a good five to ten minutes could be. She came from the school of thinking that to have a great-looking abdomen, you needed to do at least twenty minutes' worth of exercises. This is a criminal waste of time when there's so much else you could be doing. After a few months together, Cher had the strongest set of abs I'd ever come across. She gave me a good run for my money. So my real tip to you here is if you think you need to spend more time working your abs, what you probably need to be doing is improving your technique, slowing down, and making each repetition count.

Muscles worked: front of torso (rectus abdominis), sides of torso (external and internal obliques)

ABDOMINAL CURL

Setup

1. Lie on your back with feet a comfortable distance from buttocks, knees bent.
2. Place one thumb behind each ear, with fingertips touching, but not clasped, to support your head; elbows should be visible in your peripheral vision.

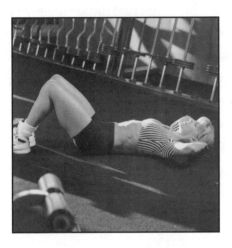 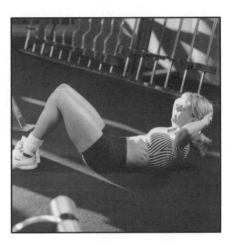

3. Contract abdominals toward spine so lower back is in contact with the floor and the pelvis is in a neutral position.

Action

1. Lift head, neck, and shoulders up in one motion to about 30 degrees or until shoulder blades clear the floor; exhale as you lift.
2. Lower torso back to starting position, making sure that your back remains in contact with the floor.
3. Take two counts to lift, counting "one thousand one," at the top of the lift, and lower in two counts.

Training tips

1. Pretend you're holding a grapefruit between your chin and your chest.
2. Don't interlock fingers and pull on head to lift yourself higher; this only strains the neck.
3. Keep pelvis in neutral alignment with buttocks relaxed; don't force a "tucked pelvis."
4. If necessary, stretch by pulling knees into chest to relieve muscle tension in lower back.

Modification

1. If you have a tight back or shortened range of motion, place feet on top of a step or lie on an incline.

Variation

1. Lie on a decline bench with hips on the high end and head at the lower end.
2. Vary arm position to vary intensity and lever length:
   a. Keep one hand behind head and extend one arm toward feet.
   b. Extend both arms above head, wrists intertwined.
   c. Hold a lightweight plate with arms crossed in front of chest.
   d. Vary the speed of both the lift and lower phases; pulse for a few counts at the top of the lift.

OBLIQUE TWIST

Setup

1. Lie on your back with left foot flat on the floor, knee bent. Lift right foot up so it's in line with your hip, and cross the ankle over the left thigh.

2. Place right hand around the back of right thigh for support, with fingers of left hand behind your head.

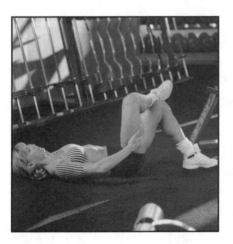 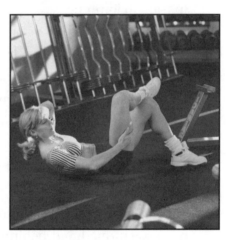

3. Contract abdominals toward your spine so low back is in contact with the floor.

Action

1. Lift head, neck, and shoulders upward in two counts, then rotate left shoulder toward right knee, keeping elbow pressed outward, but in peripheral vision.

2. As you rotate toward the right, "pin" the left hip to the floor so your hips do not move as you lift.

3. Lower torso to starting position in two counts; repeat rotation in other direction by changing arm and leg position.

Training tips

1. Keep chest open with chin off chest.
2. Lift head and neck; then twist with the shoulder so the obliques are working.
3. Lift up, then twist; don't roll from side to side on the floor.
4. With each lift, contract and "depress" abdominals toward your navel.

Variations

1. Do the same exercise on an incline or decline bench.
2. Vary the hand position, place "thigh" hand on floor instead.

REVERSE CURL

Setup
1. Lie on your back with knees drawn in toward your chest, ankles crossed with heels close to your buttocks, knees slightly open.
2. Hands are resting behind head, chest lifted.

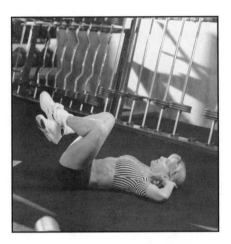 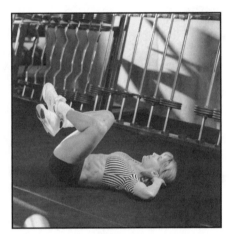

Action
1. Contract abdominals, lifting hips off the floor in two counts, about two to six inches, so knees curl in toward chest.
2. Hold, counting "one thousand one," at the top of the lift, then lower hips to the floor slowly in two counts.

Training tips
1. The lift is the result of abdominal contraction, not actively pulling the knees toward the chest.
2. Keep head and neck relaxed, with elbows on the floor.
3. Keep heels close to buttocks to help prevent legs from swinging.

Modifications

1. If it's difficult to keep arms above head, place hands beside hips (not under).
2. For a less intense version, do a reverse curl on a decline bench, so hips are higher than your head.

Variations

1. Do this same exercise on an incline bench, holding the edges of the bench behind your head.
2. For a more advanced version, do an abdominal curl at the same time, lifting head, neck, and shoulders toward knees.

STABILIZATION TECHNIQUES

After I had been teaching for a couple of years, I thought my abdominals were really strong. Then I started to experience severe back pain. I went to a physical therapist who did a number of strength tests on me. One of the tests measured my ability to stabilize my spine, using my abdominals. What we found was I was strong in the exercises I had been doing, but I had complete inability to stabilize my spine.

These next two exercises are the ones she gave me. I have used them regularly with my clients who have had similar problems and they've had remarkable success, not only in improving their posture and functional abdominal strength, but also in alleviating their pain as well.

Muscles used: abdominals, lower back (erector spinae), front of hip (iliopsoas), buttocks (gluteus maximus)

BABY LIFT

Setup

1. Lie on your back with knees bent and feet a comfortable distance from your buttocks.
2. Place hands behind head, elbows touching the floor.

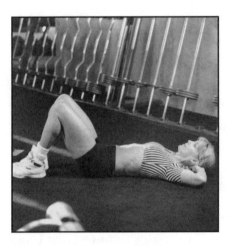 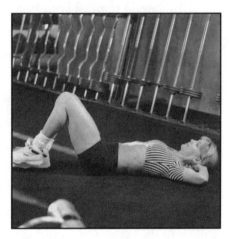

Action

1. Contract abdominals so lower back is in contact with the floor and lift one foot about an inch off the floor.
2. Continue to contract abdominals, exhale, and lift other foot off the floor.
3. Lower right foot to the floor, then the left, maintaining back contact with the floor for the entire exercise.
4. Take four counts to lift foot and four counts to lower.

Training tips

1. This exercise teaches you how to stabilize your spine and hold your pelvis in place by contracting the abdominals and holding them firmly inward while your feet move.
2. When the second leg lifts, you need to contract abdominals firmly to counteract any back arching.
3. The closer your feet are to your buttocks, the easier it is to do.
4. Only lift feet a short distance off the floor with space for a piece of paper.
5. Re-establish a neutral position with both feet on the floor before repeating exercise.

Modification

1. Lift one foot, put it down, then lift the other foot and put it down so you are alternating feet, but always have one foot on the floor for increased stabilization.

Variation

1. To make this exercise more difficult, move legs farther away from buttocks.

BRIDGING

Setup

1. Lie on your back with one leg bent and foot flat on floor, the other leg extended, foot flexed.
2. Place hands behind head, elbows open on the floor.

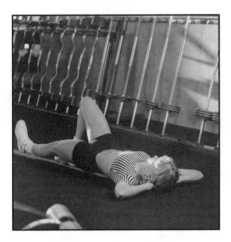 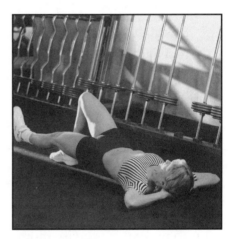

Action

1. Lift extended leg up to ankle height and hold this position.
2. Contract abdominals, keeping back in a neutral position; lift pelvis off the floor in four counts, three to five inches, so your lower back is still in neutral with only the middle back and shoulders in contact with the floor.
3. Press the heel of bent leg into the floor to help maintain position and elevate hips.
4. Lower to starting position in four counts; repeat with other leg.

Training tips

1. Keep the movement small.
2. The entire torso and extended leg should lift and lower as a unit.
3. This is a difficult exercise, and requires adequate abdominal and back strength to maintain the position.
4. Do not arch back.

Modification

1. For an easier version, do this same bridge lift with both feet on the floor or a raised step (four to six inches), legs bent.

LOWER BACK

This is one of the most neglected muscle groups in our bodies, yet it is the muscle group most frequently responsible for back pain. Therapists who specialize in spinal care have found that including exercises which strengthen the back extensors, as part of a person's overall program, is one of the most effective ways of alleviating and preventing back pain. I know for myself; no program is complete without some form of lower back work.

Don't underestimate the power and effectiveness of these exercises because they seem so subtle. They may not seem all that special or important, but if you spend a lot of time sitting or driving, they could well save you from a serious back problem in the future.

OPPOSITE ARM AND LEG LIFT

Muscles used: back extensors (erector spinae)

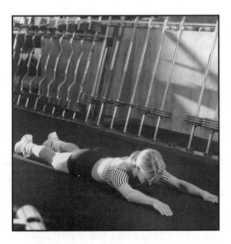 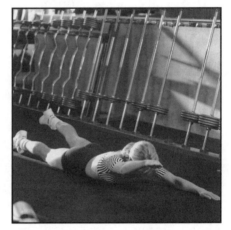

Setup

1. Lie face down with legs extended, toes touching the floor, and arms extended above head, in line with shoulders, palms down.
2. Contract abdominals slightly and pull tailbone down toward feet so your spine is in a neutral position and hips are in contact with the floor.

Action

1. Keeping head and neck aligned with the rest of your spine, lift one arm up to shoulder height and the opposite leg up to hip height in four counts.
2. Lengthen the spine by pulling arm and leg away from each other as you lift.
3. Lower to starting position in four counts and repeat, alternating with other arm and leg.

Training tips

1. Keep head down, looking just ahead of you on the floor.
2. As you lift the arm, press the shoulder blade down; the chest will slightly lift up naturally with this action.
3. Only lift leg to hip height, keeping pelvis in contact with the floor.

Variation

1. Repeat reps with same arm and leg before switching to the other side.

BACK EXTENSION

Muscles worked: lower back extensors (erector spinae), rear of thigh (hamstring), buttocks (gluteus maximus)

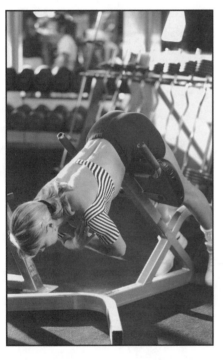 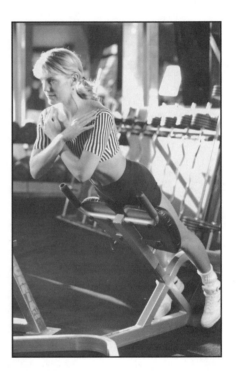

Setup

1. Lie on a hyperextension bench so hips are at the edge of pad with feet flexed underneath rests.
2. Cross arms in front of chest and lower torso down toward the floor so that you are hanging as vertically as possible; keep head and neck aligned with spine.

Action

1. Slowly lift torso upward in about eight counts until you are slightly above a parallel position.
2. Pause, counting "one thousand one" at the top of the lift while tightening buttocks; return to starting position in four counts.

Training tips

1. Don't lift so high that you overarch your spine—just above parallel is enough to strengthen your back muscles.
2. Lift up slowly; don't swing up.
3. This exercise supersets well with hamstring curls and lunges.
4. Changing arm positions changes the difficulty of the exercise.

Modification

1. If a full parallel position is too difficult, start by lifting only as high as you can, and build up to a parallel position.

Variation

1. Change arm positions so hands are behind head, behind back (easiest), or with elbows lifted to side (most difficult).

Notes

Notes

Notes

ELEVEN

The Big
E-Z Stretch

STRETCH

*To grow, to expand or extend
beyond normal limits
through an unbroken period
of time.*
—Random House Dictionary

What do a hot bath and stretching have in common? They both relax your muscles. I think I never would have gotten fit if it weren't for Epsom salts and a good hot bath. While I don't recommend that you jump into a hot tub right after a heavy-duty sweating session, though, you do want to take the time to stretch.

After a workout, when your muscles are really warm, is the perfect time to elongate muscles, increase joint flexibility, and just plain relax. Fitness benefits aside, stretching can help you tune out the environment and tune in to you. Once I learned to quiet my muscles, breathe with my own bodily rhythms, and release muscle tension, I learned to quiet my mind as well, creating an enormous sense of well-being and mental restfulness.

If burning calories is number one on your fitness list, don't negate this reposeful state as a waste of time. Stretching can help you learn how to handle the stress which may cause overeating and other roadblocks in your life. This is important to maintaining permanent weight loss. I found this to be particularly true for myself.

In my work with Cher, she was *the* aerobic diva. Her primary focus was on pushing her limits and burning megacalories. However, as hard as she worked out, Cher found finishing her workout with a long, slow, relaxing stretch and a guided visual gave her a sense of relaxation and completeness, which really enabled her to go out and face her incredibly demanding lifestyle. This encouraged me to regularly include this in my own personal training schedule.

Stretching: A Natural Analgesic

Here's a common scenario: You're stressed; your mind is screaming to relax on command, which of course it can't. As you get more uptight, your muscles become more tense. Now you have a headache that runs from the top of your head to your toes. You wish it was the weekend so you could "relax," but it's only Wednesday. The high you felt from an aerobics class that morning was a short-term fix. Does this sound all too familiar? Unfortunately, too many of us can relate; I know I can. We expend a lot of energy trying desperately to break loose from this rat-race routine. While stretching isn't the end-all nirvana, it can provide a daily escape to give you some physical and mental relief if you do it diligently. It works for me.

Taking a mental vacation on a daily basis just by stretching seems far too easy, doesn't it? Most of the experts I talked to agree, however, that stretching, coupled with correct breathing and visualization, can positively alter our neurological response to stress. Focusing your full attention on how your body feels, being aware of muscle sensations, and concentrating on your movements will help release those tension "holding patterns" in your muscles, so your body will feel more relaxed, too.

When I do daily meditations, I handle the regular stress of my life with a greater degree of clarity and calm. Plus, I have a better night's sleep because my muscles aren't carrying nearly as much tension. The ability to refocus on yourself and not on the events of the day does take some practice. But with a little effort, you'd be surprised how easily both your mind and your muscles will respond.

Why Stretch?

Relaxation at the tip of your fingers sounds great, but what else can stretching do for you? For one thing, stretching increases your flexibility; along with cardiovascular and strength training, it's one of the basics of any complete fitness program. The ability to move with a freer and greater range of motion lets your muscles be more supple, or "elastic," so they can respond to daily activity with less potential for injury.

When you're stiff or inflexible, your posture might also suffer because some muscles have to do the work of others that aren't strong or limber enough, which in turn pulls on your joints. You know the feeling; you try to lift your leg up, and it feels like the muscles in the back of your leg are holding you down. When your muscles and joints are more supple, you'll move easier and faster, with less effort; your limbs won't feel quite so heavy because they're not fighting tension.

Susan Dey insists that regular stretching has virtually made a chronic sciatic problem disappear. "After you do a workout, for some reason the one thing you want to cheat yourself on is the stretching afterward, because you say, 'Oh, I've done my workout so I'm not going to stretch … I'm going to hurry,' " she told me. "But the stretching part is as important as building up a muscle. After years of dealing with sciatica, I have learned that after I exercise, if I do stretching exercises which only take a few minutes, I don't have a sciatica problem anymore. When I get a sciatica problem and when I think it through, I will find out that the last couple of times that I worked really, really hard, I forgot to stretch or decided not to."

Making stretching a consistent habit can improve the overall quality of muscle function. If they're more flexible, your muscles will respond by contracting faster and with greater efficiency to the demands of sports and other vigorous activities. Consistent stretching becomes even more important as you grow older. Remember the old saying, "Use it, or lose it"? If you're not as flexible as you used to be, age isn't the culprit. You don't lose the ability to be flexible as you get older (or any other form of fitness), it's just necessary to include stretching on a regular basis to maintain it.

I had an older gentleman client, sixty-four, who came to me with a degenerative condition in his hip. He'd lost about a half-inch of bone and was in continual pain in his back and neck. Along with muscle imbalances, his body was twisted in tightness. He hadn't stretched in years, although he had worked out all of his life. Along with strength work, I put him on a very aggressive stretching program—he never skipped it—and spent a lot of time recreating flexibility so he could walk. Stretching was one of the most important components of his program.

After a few months, he noticed a really significant change. He was standing straight and was pain-free for the first time in years. He was so used to living with back pain, that after a while he just adapted. He hadn't realized how bad it really was until he got rid of it. Now, he practices his stretches regularly. I ended up training this man for four years; he was amazing. Just know a minimum of five minutes a day is definitely an easy way to ensure healthy, stress-free joints and a lifetime of mobility and agility.

When to Stretch

You can and should stretch daily, especially on those off-workout days. Once you're out of bed in the morning and moving, muscles become imbalanced from the natural push and pull of everyday tasks. However, your muscles elongate and become more flexible as the day wears on. Even a more active lifestyle doesn't really provide enough stretching and muscular relaxation to achieve flexibility necessary to keep muscles healthy.

I'm really fit and active, and have been for the last eight years, although I suffered from a chronic back problem caused by tightness. My chiropractor, Dr. Arnold Sandlow, gave me a series of stretches I do every day before I even get out of bed. Many of these are included in the stretch series in this chapter. I find these help me remain pain-free.

Stretching feels great when done correctly, and anyone can learn to stretch, regardless of body type or age. While you can stretch anytime, anyplace, it's really important to stretch *when you've finished your workout.* When you're warm from activity, your muscles are most receptive to lengthening. Once you're completely "cooled down" again, muscles and the connective tissue around the joints tend to tighten back up and become more rigid, thus less pliable.

Optimally, you should stretch for twenty to thirty minutes, three times to five times a week. If you're on a time budget, at the very least allow yourself five to ten minutes at the end of your training session to stretch the major muscles that you just worked out. Although it's a short time period, concentration and attitude can also induce a relaxed state of mind.

How to Stretch

Knowing how to stretch correctly makes stretching easier. For starters, here are a few tips:

1. Get comfortable. Wear loose-fitting clothing that allows you freedom to move.

2. Choose a place where you won't be interrupted so you can really relax and focus on your muscles.

3. Put on some of your favorite "soft" music, if this helps you.

The stretching exercises I chose for this chapter are some of my favorite stretches. I've put them into a short routine, so you should do them in the order shown for the greatest relaxation and muscle release. Feel free to pick and choose any exercises that you like and that feel good. However, you should always start with exercise No. 1—lying on your back, with arms and legs relaxed; this will help get you into what I call the "stretch mode." This feeling is similar to how you feel just before you fall asleep, when you're drifting. Close your eyes and try to clear your mind by concentrating on your breathing for a minute or two. Allow your breathing to become slow and rhythmic. Once your attention is focused, you'll become more aware of body sensations as you do each stretch.

Achieving the Big E-Z Stretch

For each stretch in your program, follow these guidelines:

1. **Go E-Z.** Only stretch to the point of mild tension. At this point, stop and hold the stretch for at least thirty seconds or more. As the muscle relaxes, the tension you felt will subside, and you can move a little deeper into the stretch, holding it for a little longer, up to one or two minutes depending upon your comfort level. To increase flexibility, you need to move slowly.

2. **Breathe naturally and rhythmically.** Inhale as you begin to stretch and slowly exhale as you move into each stretch position. Continue to breathe as you hold and deepen each stretch, relaxing and releasing tension throughout the entire body.

3. **Do not bounce.** Hold each stretch without a lot of movement, except to increase or decrease constant tension on the muscle you're stretching. Don't bounce or pulse through the stretch. Bouncing places stress on the muscle, causing it to contract—not relax—which defeats the purpose.

4. **Feel where you are stretching.** You should feel the stretch in the belly or center of the muscle, not at your joints. If you feel strange sensations around your joints, you could be placing strain on your ligaments and connective tissue. In this case, recheck your alignment and make sure you're in the correct position. If you feel sensations elsewhere in your body, be conscious of the feeling, letting your attention focus on it and letting it go.

5. **Know your own limits.** Stretching beyond your boundaries could be more harmful than helpful. Tight muscles or stiff joints can make stretching uncomfortable at first. If you feel too much

tension or muscular trembling, ease off a bit, and increase the amount of tension gradually. Above all else, stop if it hurts. When I first started teaching aerobics, I tore both my hamstrings by overstretching because I never understood that stretching didn't have to hurt to be effective. Never stretch to the limit of pain.

6. **Flexibility is joint specific.** Not all joints were created equal; range of motion can differ between upper and lower body. For example, your shoulders might be more flexible than your hips. Or, one shoulder joint can be more flexible than the other. Although you can't change your structure, you can stretch to increase your flexibility potential, so consider each joint separately as you stretch; zero in mentally so that you can be aware of telltale signs and adapt accordingly.

7. **Flexibility varies.** How you feel, how tense you are, the weather, and how your muscles respond can vary from day to day. Check in with your body before you start and adapt according to how you feel that day. Avoid expecting too much. Sometimes taking it a little easier is what your body is asking for. I find in particular, after I've had a hard workout, or if the weather is cold, I'm much tighter than usual and it takes me a little longer to get into a deep stretch.

8. **Maintain alignment.** Maintaining correct alignment while stretching is one of my "bug-bears." I'm insistent with my clients; it's not how deep you go in the stretch, it's about correct form. Proper body alignment is crucial to gaining flexibility. Always stretch a muscle in the direction the muscle fibers run in; choose a position that's easy to maintain so your concentration is on the muscle you're stretching, not on the difficulty of the position.

∾

SPIRIT
Spiritual nourishment feeds the heart.
—Unknown

∾

Tuning in and Letting Go

Stretching for flexibility is one thing, stretching and relaxing is another. While the two go hand in hand, relaxing by command alone takes some practice. Susan Dey and I were stretching after her workout one day, and she reminded me how difficult it was to give in and relax when she had so much to do. She said, "Stretching is so important because it's my transition period … It's so hard to make myself go and spend the time. I have lists and lists of things I'm supposed to be doing and I always feel torn apart. If I'm exercising, I can't do any of these things I'm supposed to do. It would take a commitment (for me) just to say, 'No, I'm going to exercise first.'

"So I'd focus on the exercising and then at the end of that period of time, when I do my stretching, part of my breathing in and breathing out is mentally saying to myself, 'Yes, yes, how good you are.' I also prepare myself, now I am ready to tackle my lists; now I can go about the rest of my day." Susan discovered very quickly how important both stretching and mental permission to "float" was to her entire well-being.

The most important tool you can use to guide you is your breath. Deep breathing (or belly breathing), involves breathing with the diaphragm. When you put a hand on your abdomen while inhaling, you'll feel the diaphragm expand your belly; when you exhale slowly and smoothly, your belly pulls inward toward your spine. Deep breathing gently through each stretch will increase your focus on yourself, letting you slip into deep relaxation.

To Tune in:

1. Concentrate first on observing your breathing. Notice how your body feels as you inhale and exhale. Focus on the flow of your breath and the sensation of breathing deeper than normally.

2. Be aware of any body sensations as you move into a stretch, as you hold the stretch, and as the muscle releases.

3. Keep your mind focused and present. Don't let your mind wander and think about stressful things, you'll have plenty of time for that later. Bring your attention back by concentrating on the evenness of your breath.

4. Breathe out slowly as you reach the tension point of each stretch and continue to breathe deeply through the exercise.

To Let go:

1. As your muscles relax, allow yourself to "sink" into each stretch, feeling your body release tension.

2. Visualize each muscle in your mind as you're stretching: where it's situated, what it looks like as the muscle fibers elongate. Imagine your muscles lengthening.

3. Continue to pay attention to bodily signs and the sensations that accompany each stretch; then release.

My Twenty-Step Relaxation Plan

Directions: For a complete stretching program, do these exercises in the order listed. Follow the stretching guidelines discussed in this chapter. You'll need a towel for some of the exercises. If you're short on time, choose exercises for the tightest and most inflexible muscles; hamstrings and lower back, in particular, are notorious stress offenders. To really get the most benefit from these exercises, read the tuning in/letting go tips at the end of each caption. If you're new to stretching, these will help you focus and stay in the moment. Enjoy!

1   LONG-LYING STRETCH

Muscles stretched: front of shoulders (anterior deltoid), chest (pectoralis major), abdominals (rectus abdominis), and hip flexors (iliopsoas)

Setup

1. Lie on your back, legs straight, with arms extended overhead, close to ears, and elbows relaxed.
2. Tilt tailbone so your pelvis is in a neutral position, maintaining your spine's natural arch.

Action

1. Squeeze shoulder blades, pressing them to the floor so your shoulders drop; straighten arms, reaching overhead; exhale.
2. At the same time, point your toes and stretch your torso so it feels like you're being pulled at either end of your body.
3. Don't overarch your spine; maintain neutral even though your lower back is lifted slightly off the floor.

Tuning in / Letting go

1. Be aware of any tension you might feel throughout your chest, shoulder, or abdominals region.
2. Feel your shoulders relaxing toward the floor as you stretch your arms overhead.
3. Notice all of the points where your body touches the floor: neck shoulders, back, buttocks, thighs, calves. How does the floor support you?
4. Let your body feel like it's floating on a bed of feathers as you release the stretch into the floor.

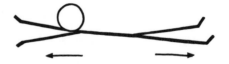

2 NECK STRETCH

Muscles stretched: neck (sternocleidomastoid and levator scapula) and upper back (trapezius)

Setup
1. Lie on your back with knees bent and feet a comfortable distance from your buttocks.
2. Place hands behind head, fingertips touching, elbows open.
3. Contract abdominals so your spine is in a neutral position and your back is in contact with the floor.

Action
1. Bring elbows forward, close to ears, exhale, and drop chin toward your chest so shoulders leave the floor.

Tuning in / Letting go
1. Close your eyes and feel the gentle pull on the back of your neck and upper back.
2. Be aware of any tension in your shoulders as you drop your chin.
3. Notice how light your head feels in your hands as you begin to relax.
4. "Give in" to the stretch, letting your chin drop all the way to your chest, without fighting to lift your head back up.

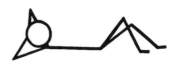

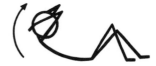

3 HIP-FLEXOR STRETCH

Muscles stretched: front of hips (iliopsoas) and buttocks (gluteus maximus)

Setup

1. Lie on your back with left leg straight, toes relaxed; right leg is bent in toward chest with your hands behind the thigh.
2. Head, neck, and shoulders are relaxed with lower back in contact with the floor.

Action

1. Gently pull right knee toward chest, begin to exhale, pushing through heel of left leg until you feel a stretch in the front of your thigh.
2. Keep lower back, hips, and left calf in contact with the floor.
3. As tension releases, bring knee a little closer to chest, feeling a stretch in your buttocks.
4. Keep neck and shoulders relaxed and on the floor; don't hunch your shoulders or pull on your leg.

Tuning in / Letting go

1. Feel the straight leg lengthen, "opening" and flattening the front of your hip.
2. Notice how your bent leg seems weightless against your chest as you continue to breathe and exhale.

(NOTE: Do stretches 3 through 6 in order, using the same leg. Then switch and do the same sequence using the other leg.)

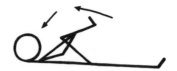

4 SPINAL TWIST

Muscles stretched: front of shoulders (anterior deltoid), abdominals (rectus abdominis, obliques), middle back (latissimus dorsi), upper hip (gluteus medius), and buttocks (gluteus maximus)

Setup

1. From the stretch No. 3 position, keep right knee in toward chest, place left hand on the outside of right knee; extend right arm to the side at shoulder height, palm down.

Action

1. Keep shoulders on the floor, exhale, and slowly press right knee across your body's midline toward the floor.
2. Don't force or push your knee down; let hip follow naturally as tension subsides.
3. Return to starting position by lifting knee first, then rolling back to center.

Tuning in / Letting go

1. Feel if any tightness in your hip or torso restricts your twisting motion.
2. Feel the knee go lower to the floor, without force, but with control.
3. Let your shoulders and upper back support your body against the floor.
4. Feel your spine lengthen as your knee continues to drop and your hip relaxes.

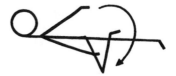

5   PRETZEL

Muscles stretched: buttocks (gluteus maximus), hips (gluteus medius), and lower back (erector spinae)

Setup
1. From stretch No. 4, bend left knee and place foot on floor; right knee is still bent in toward chest.
2. Cross right heel over left thigh, so right hip is slightly turned out.
3. Place a towel behind your left thigh and hold either end with palms facing your body, with a slight tension on the towel.
4. Head and neck are relaxed with shoulders touching the floor.

Action
1. Lift left foot off floor; using the towel, exhale, and pull knees in toward chest until you feel a stretch in your buttocks and hips.
2. Slowly return legs to the floor, letting the towel support you all the way down.

Tuning in / Letting go
1. Notice the tension releasing in your hip socket of the leg that's crossed.
2. Notice as you relax that your legs feel "lighter," and you're no longer dependent on the towel to maintain the stretch.
3. Feel your buttocks relax and lower back lengthen against the floor.

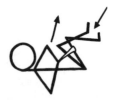

6   HAMSTRING STRETCH

Muscles stretched: rear of thigh (hamstring)

Setup

1. From stretch No. 5, bend right knee into chest and place towel behind ankle.
2. Hold the towel with some tension on it with both hands, palms facing in; then straighten right leg in the air, foot flexed.
3. Keep left knee bent and foot flat on floor a comfortable distance from buttocks.
4. Contract abdominals so lower back is touching the floor.

Action

1. Using the towel, exhale and gently pull right leg toward chest, keeping it as straight as possible.
2. Keep foot flexed.
3. Gently hold the towel with elbows slightly bent; don't "hang on" to the towel, contracting neck and shoulder muscles.
4. Bend knee in toward chest before returning foot to the floor.

Tuning in / Letting go

1. Feel your leg being supported by the towel.
2. As the tension in the rear of your leg relaxes, the rest of your body will relax too.
3. Focus on your breathing, tension dissipating with each breath.

(Do this same series of stretches, numbers 3 through 6, with the left leg.)

7 ROCK AND ROLL

Muscles stretched: lower back (erector spinae), buttocks (gluteus maximus)

Setup

1. Lie on your back with both knees bent at a 90-degree angle to your hips.
2. Place one hand behind each thigh, elbows relaxed.
3. Keep head, neck, and shoulders relaxed and in contact with the floor.

Action

1. Contract abdominals, exhale, and slowly pull knees in toward chest until hips lift slightly off floor; keep head and neck aligned.
2. Hold the position; then rock gently back and forth on your lower back and tailbone, like a massaging motion a few times, then relax back into the stretch, keeping knees toward chest.

Tuning in / Letting go

1. Close your eyes; let your legs feel buoyant.
2. Feel your spine against the floor; then imagine descending downward, through the floor, tension leaving your body as you rock.

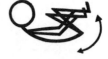

8   INNER-THIGH STRETCH

Muscles stretched: inner thighs (adductors)

Setup
1. Lie on your back, hands behind head, and place soles of your feet together; turn knees outward.
2. Contract abdominals so pelvis is in neutral alignment with lower back in contact with the floor.

Action
1. Exhale and let knees slowly "fall" open naturally toward the floor, keeping lower back in contact with the floor the entire time.
2. Make sure feet are far enough in front of you to maintain alignment without feeling strained.
3. Let upper torso relax, so the concentration of the stretch is through the inner thighs.

Tuning in / Letting go
1. Notice if your legs resist the downward pull of gravity as your knees open.
2. Each time you exhale, contract abdominals through your spine to send your breath out your back and through the floor.
3. Feel yourself "sinking" into the floor with each breath as your legs continue to relax.

9 SIDE-LYING QUAD STRETCH

Muscles stretched: front of thighs (quadriceps), hip flexors (iliopsoas)

Setup

1. Lie on your left side, head resting on upper arm; extend both legs in line with your torso, with knees bent and stacked on top of each other.
2. Wrap a towel around the front of your right ankle, and hold it with your right hand.
3. Contract abdominals to keep pelvis in a neutral position and body in one straight line.

Action

1. Lift right leg a few inches above left; keep knee facing forward and gently apply tension on the towel; pull right heel back toward buttocks. You'll feel a stretch in the front of your hip and thigh.
2. Keep legs parallel and stacked, even though right leg is lifted.
3. Don't pull so hard on the towel that it causes your back to arch; maintain a neutral position.

Tuning in / Letting go

1. Feel the front of your leg lengthen as tension releases; after you stretch both thighs, your legs will feel longer, you'll feel taller.
2. Notice how easy it is to lose balance if you pull too hard on the towel; be gentle as you stretch and let your other muscles support you.

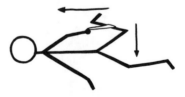

10 MODIFIED COBRA

Muscles stretched: abdominals (rectus abdominis), chest (pectoralis major)

Setup
1. Lie facedown, legs extended, with elbows bent close to your sides, forearms and palms on the floor.
2. Head and neck are aligned with the rest of your spine; contract abdominals so hipbones are in contact with the floor so there is minimal arch in lower back.

Action
1. Press upward onto your hands so your chest and head are off the floor, and you're supported on your forearms; exhale.
2. Lift up only high enough to feel a mild stretch through the front of your torso; keep elbows in contact with the floor.

Tuning in / Letting go
1. As you exhale, feel the tension leave your neck and shoulders as you press your shoulder blades down and back.
2. Notice the weight of your head as you hold yourself upright.
3. As you relax, create as much space as possible between your ears and your shoulders.
4. Feel your breathing against the floor as your abdominals expand and contract.

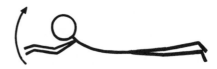

11 CAT STRETCH

Muscles stretched: back muscles (erector spinae, trapezius, rhomboids)

Setup
1. Kneel on all fours so knees are aligned under hips and hands are just in front of shoulders, arms extended with elbows slightly bent.
2. Back is flat and head, neck, spine, and tailbone are all aligned.

Action
1. Inhale and round back up like a cat; let head drop and follow the natural extension of the spine.
2. Exhale and slowly return to starting position, elongating spine as you do.

Tuning in / Letting go
1. Feel the position of each vertebrae as you round your back; feel the space between your vertebrae; feel the spine lengthening between your vertebrae as you continue to hold the stretch.
2. Let your head feel heavy and hang.
3. As you round, visualize the bottom tips of your shoulder blades separating, creating a wide space in the center of your back.
4. As you return to the starting position, feel the tips of your shoulder blades pull together as though magnets were attached to them, pulling your body back to a straight line.

12 SIT-BACK STRETCH

Muscles stretched: chest (pectoralis major), front, middle, and rear shoulder (anterior, medial, and posterior deltoid), arms (biceps)

Setup

1. Kneel on the floor with your knees separated under your hips, arms extended in front of you, shoulder distance apart.
2. Head and neck are aligned and you're looking at the floor.

Action

1. "Sit back" to bring buttocks toward your heels; walk your fingertips forward, exhale, and press chest toward the floor.

Tuning in / Letting go

1. Feel your shoulder blades separate, expanding the space between them.
2. Each time you exhale, feel the weightlessness of your body, inducing a sense of submergence into the floor with your chest and arms.

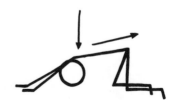

13 SHIN-AND-CALF STRETCH

Muscles stretched: front and rear of the lower leg (tibialis anterior and soleus)

Setup

1. Kneel with buttocks close to the floor so one foot is flat on the floor, leg bent; the other leg is bent so the front of the shin is on the floor.
2. Place both hands on the floor in front of you, back is straight with abdominals contracted and rib cage lifted.

Action

1. Exhale, and press body weight downward through the buttocks and forward through the shoulders; you'll feel a stretch in the rear of the heel that's on the floor and in the front of the shin.
2. Don't "sit" on your back heel as this places too much stress on the knee.

Tuning in / Letting go

1. Feel the slight pulling sensation in the rear of your heel as you stretch; be aware of the pressure on the bottom of your foot as it contacts the floor.
2. Try to wiggle your toes; if your body weight is too far forward, this will be difficult; shift your body weight into your heel, if necessary.
3. Notice any tension in your knees or back while holding this position; let it go as you exhale.

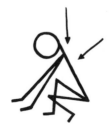

14 "TUCKED" HIP STRETCH

Muscles stretched: hip flexors (iliopsoas) and front of thigh (quadriceps)

Setup

1. Kneel on one leg with knee under hip and top of foot flat on floor; the other leg is out in front of you, knee bent to a 90-degree angle over the ankle.
2. Place hands on thighs for support, contract abdominals, and lift rib cage.
3. Your back should be in a neutral position, with tailbone pointing to the floor.

Action

1. Maintain position, exhale, and tuck the bottom part of your pelvis forward until you feel the front of your hip lengthen and stretch.

Tuning in / Letting go

1. Try to move only in your pelvic region, so the rest of your body is stationary.
2. Imagine your hip muscles relaxing their hold on your pelvis so that you can move freely in a forward and back motion.

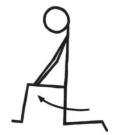

15 RUNNER'S STRETCH

Muscles stretched: hip flexors (iliopsoas), front of thigh (quadriceps), and buttocks (gluteus maximus)

Setup

1. This is a difficult position if you're inflexible. If you can't place your hand comfortably on the floor, do the same stretch in a standing lunge position.
2. From stretch no. 14, keep front leg bent and in line with ankle; place opposite hand on the floor, close to your foot, and maintain support hand on thigh.
3. Extend kneeling leg behind you so that it's straight and your body weight is supported on your toes.
4. Keep back straight, maintaining a straight line from head to foot of extended leg.

Action

1. Maintain alignment and front leg position; exhale and press hips toward the floor, bending knee slightly until you feel a stretch in the front of your hips.

Tuning in / Letting go

1. As your hips drop, feel as if you're pressing against an imaginary wall as your torso lengthens.
2. As you stretch, feel the pressure drop away from your pelvis.

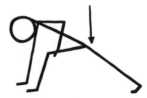

16 OVERHEAD STRETCH

Muscles stretched: chest (pectoralis major), front of shoulders (anterior deltoid), and abdominals (rectus abdominis)

Setup
1. Stand with feet hip-width apart, knees slightly bent, and tailbone pointing to the floor.
2. Hold a towel in front of your thighs, one end in each hand, palms facing thighs.
3. Contract abdominals, lift rib cage, and relax shoulders.

Action
1. Lift arms overhead, a little wider than shoulder-width apart; without arching lower back, exhale and press arms to the rear until you feel a stretch in the chest area.
2. Keep arms straight, but not locked, and maintain a slight tension on the towel.

Tuning in / Letting go
1. Close your eyes; visualize your shoulder blades traveling downward until the lower tips touch.
2. As your shoulder blades drop, so do your shoulders.
3. Let your arms feel weightless, but supported by your body.
4. Feel the floor with your feet and the firmness of your support.

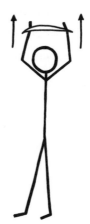

17 TRICEPS TOWEL STRETCH

Muscles stretched: rear of upper arm (triceps) and front of shoulders (anterior deltoid)

Setup

1. Stand with feet hip-width apart, knees slightly bent, and tailbone pointing to the floor; arms relaxed.
2. Contract abdominals, lift rib cage, and relax shoulders.
3. Hold the end of a towel with one hand; place the same hand on your shoulder so elbow is pointing forward and other end of the towel is down your back, thumb down.
4. Grasp the other end of the towel with your other hand, thumb up and close to your waist; walk hand up towel to place slight tension on it.

Action

1. Maintain standing position and pull down on the towel, lifting arm so elbow points toward the ceiling.
2. Keep arm being stretched close to your ear, shoulders relaxed.

Tuning in / Letting go

1. Visualize your arm being lifted and pulled upward by a string attached to your elbow.
2. Feel the lengthening of the triceps as you pull downward on the towel.

18 OVERHEAD REACH

Muscles stretched: middle back (latissimus dorsi), sides of torso (obliques)

Setup

1. Stand with legs wider than shoulder-width apart, feet turned out slightly, with one knee bent to a 90-degree angle, the other leg straight.
2. Contract abdominals and lift rib cage.
3. Place one hand on thigh of bent knee for support and extend the opposite arm in the air, close to your ear.

Action

1. Maintain lower-body position and slowly lean toward bent leg so arm above head and straight leg form a diagonal line, and you feel a stretch in the side of your torso.
2. Don't lean so far sideways that you throw your hip out to the side and lose alignment.
3. Avoid slouching or bending the torso sideways, and keep rib cage lifted and abdominals contracted.

Tuning in / Letting go

1. As you elongate and stretch, feel the shoulder blade drop down and back, creating more space between your ear and shoulder.
2. As you lean, notice how the muscles in your torso support you from falling over sideways like a rag doll.

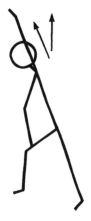

19 SIDE TO SIDE

Muscles stretched: neck (levator scapula) and upper back (trapezius)

Setup

1. Stand erect with feet hip-width apart, knees bent, pelvis in good alignment, with arms relaxed by your sides.
2. Contract abdominals, drop shoulders down and back, and look straight ahead.

Action

1. Slowly bring one ear toward shoulder, keeping shoulders down and maintaining body alignment, while you elongate your neck muscles; don't lift shoulder toward ear.

Tuning in / Letting go

1. Close your eyes; let the weight of your head dropping to your shoulder stretch the opposite side of your neck.
2. Notice your breathing and how it helps to release all tension in your neck and shoulders.

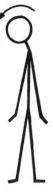

20 THE BIG LAT/SPINE STRETCH

Muscles stretched: back muscles (trapezius, rhomboids, latissimus dorsi), middle and rear shoulders (medial and posterior deltoids), buttocks (gluteus maximus)

Setup

1. Stand and face a sturdy support (such as a pole, door, or sink counter) with feet a little wider than hip-width apart, knees slightly bent, abdominals contracted, and tailbone pointing down.
2. Extend both arms in front of you at chest height and grasp the support with both hands, shoulders down and back.

Action

1. Bend knees and tuck tailbone under as you sit back so your body weight is toward your heels, allowing your back to round like the letter C, and open your shoulder blades.
2. Drop chin so that head and neck follow the natural curve of spine as you stretch.
3. Pull back away from support to increase stretch.
4. Keep abdominals contracted, so back can round and stretch.

Tuning in / Letting go

1. Feel your back muscles expanding, like butterfly wings, as if they were pushing out of your skin.
2. Feel the lengthening of your spine between the vertebrae as you continue to stretch.
3. Notice any holding pattern or uncomfortable area in your back; focus on the spot, making it smaller and smaller in your mind until it disappears.

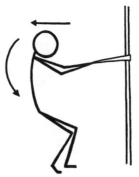

Notes

Notes

Notes

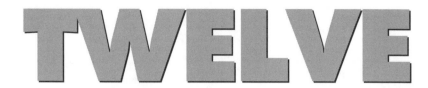

TWELVE

Maintaining, Reassessing, & Retesting

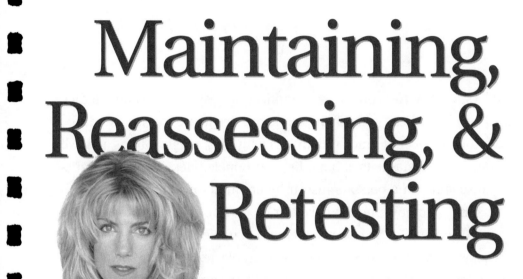

To keep a lamp burning, we
have to keep putting oil in it.
—Mother Teresa

t's so easy to want instant gratification, especially when we face ourselves head-on. When people are desperate for an instant fix, the prospect of quick weight loss with pills, magic lotions, passive exercise, or insta-diets is hope beyond hopelessness. Advertisements that scheme on a person's insecurity are ludicrous, of course, but it's become a lucrative moneymaker for those who prey on potential customers looking for an easier, softer way. It makes me so angry because it plays right into people's most vulnerable tendencies. It would be wonderful to take a pill, go to sleep, and have every bit of unwanted fat melt away in the night, but the truth is, it's a lie disguised as a miracle.

Don't Leave Before the Miracle

Anyone who's ever exercised regularly knows that it takes time, effort, and consistency to reap the benefits of an exercise program. If you drop out before your body has had time to acclimate, you're missing out on all the "good stuff" that comes between the lines.

Getting and staying in shape belongs in a much bigger picture. It's beyond your body; it's about your self-worth, which grows as you continue to support your own efforts by exercising. It's finding the strength within, not just physically, to hang in there and exercise the next time, and the next time, and the next. It's the most loving and disciplined way to improve your self-esteem. It's a form of self-assertion that we learn on the most primary levels. We learn to stick up for ourselves beyond the stresses of our daily lives by learning first to physically assert ourselves.

One morning, when Anita and I were working out together, she said the most wonderful thing: "When you're physically fit and strong, you're better prepared for stress. To handle stress requires that you confront whatever is the source—people, places, or circumstances, and that takes strength."

I think of it like this: We resign from the debating society that tells us "I can't," "I'm too tired," "It'll never work for me," "I don't have time," "I don't feel like it." Turning away from that mode of surrender, we can get into some serious, positive action. As a result, we go out into the world with a truly greater sense of strength, which manifests itself both physically and mentally.

This strength is cyclical and fuels us to keep going, to want to continue to change. It helps us build an internal support system by giving us warning signals and picking us up when we fall—fall into an exercise rut, fall into compulsive eating, or fall out of sync with ourselves. What's most difficult about change is allowing some breathing room so life isn't always so absolute. This is the gray area—the hardest place in which to be. It's easier to have things be black and white: I'm on a diet, or I'm not; I'm in shape, or I'm not. It's either *all* good or *all* bad; a perfectionistic attitude goes against our own instinctive human nature to be in constant ebb and flow.

∽

*The growth of understanding follows an ascending spiral rather than
a straight one.*
—*Joanna Field,* Each Day a New Beginning

If you expect yourself to perfectly follow any nutrition or exercise plan
all the time, you're set up to drop out. Watch out for an all-or-nothing
mentality; it's a trap to chain you to permanent procrastination or
burning out. It's also a "now I've blown it" attitude which sets us up to
eat the whole bag of Doritos . . . with the guacamole. This rationaliza-
tion becomes: "So now I might as well eat whatever I want and start
again next week."

You can easily talk yourself out of exercising, too, when your inner
voice argues, "I've missed three days in a row, so I'll start back next
week." A missed day becomes next week and usually passes right into
another week, then a month. Before you know it, you're back to poor
eating habits and vegetating on the couch.

∽

*You can't think yourself into right actions,
but you can act yourself into right thinking. All it takes is the
willingness to try one day at a time.*
—*Keli Roberts*

Changing within Reason

If you've set sky-high goals that you're having trouble sticking to regularly, you might be biting off more than you can chew. I've seen my
clients have *more* success doing *less* and taking comfortable baby steps

than other individuals who have tried to do everything at peak level all at once. Setting a pace that you can handle can protect you from "deprivation backlash." Make sure you're really comfortable with your "change boundaries," so that you don't overstep them. Otherwise, you might burn out and drop out.

If you do "drop out" (I like to think of it more as "slip off" or wandering), you don't have to wait for the new year to start a resolution. Just do it *now*, instead of next week or next month. Rather than backing out, back up and re-evaluate what your life requires of you *today*. In chapter 4, you designed a personal weekly program. Remember how I advised you to chart only one week at a time? That's because unplanned commitments sometimes pop out of nowhere and "seem" to sabotage the very organized schedule that you planned to follow. Maybe your time availability has changed, work or family demands are higher, or your goals need some revamping. Just like the seasons, life changes in an unfaltering, reoccurring cycle; be adaptable so that you can continue to be successful.

There's a fine line we walk in terms of change. How much is enough, or what's too little? If you feel you've hit a plateau, either in your diet or exercise program so that you're not continuing to see the changes you want (or if you're overwhelmed with the whole process), I suggest that you go back to chapter 1 and check those areas of your life in which you're willing to plunge or wade. Perhaps there's an issue that you're wading through that you need to dive into, boots and all ... just plunge. Maybe you're trying to do too much and are feeling defeated by it all; it seems overwhelming to think of maintaining fitness for a month or two, let alone a lifetime.

Just remember the baby step concept. If you can do it for today, but are panicking about keeping it up for the rest of your life, you need to concentrate on doing it one day at a time. Forever is a scary word, but forever will get there one step at a time. What you need to remind yourself is that what was difficult today will get easier tomorrow; then the thought of a lifetime doesn't seem so unmanageable.

On the other hand, if it's too much for you to handle today, then easy does it, look at your priorities, and perhaps restructure, because it might really be too much.

Honest Evaluation

If your body is being stubborn and won't budge from a certain weight, your plateau might be food related. Take a look at "Baby Steps, Big Changes" in chapter 3; see if you've fully cut back the foods that sabotage you and added the ones that will change you. Or go back to your food exchanges and see if you've been cheating on your portions; honest eating isn't easy. You might have to go back to precisely measuring your exchange amounts to get you back on track.

Whether it's exercise or diet, your body responds best to a little surprise. Your body gets bored and stops functioning optimally in the same way your mind gets bored when it isn't stimulated. The saying "variety is the spice of life" is certainly the case in point here. So now is the time to: try different foods within the exchange lists, bike instead of run, do your strength-training exercises back to front (if you *always* do squats before lunges, do your lunges first or do your upper body before your lower body), or vary the intensity of your workout. Your body is *stimulated* by change. If you stick to the same program for months, your body will let you know by coming to a stop and plateauing. It's body language for "give me something new and exciting to do!"

Sometimes what seems like a plateau is more like a resting point. There might be any number of reasons why your body is hanging on to it's old shape. Keeping an honest account of your workout and nutritional habits will give you perspective. The body doesn't change overnight; it's a slow process. If you're overanxious—for example, you weigh yourself ten times a day, looking for a change on the scale, or you stare in the mirror constantly looking for a change in your clothes—you're going to be disappointed. Your body will respond, but it truly is gradual. When you started exercising, it was a slower process, but then you got stronger over a period of time. Reprogramming your body to continue to respond is the same gradual process.

I love gardening; it gives me real peace of mind. But when I plant flowers from seeds, I notice my impatience while waiting for them to sprout, grow leaves, grow tall, and then flower. If every day I bent down and studied the growth to see if anything had happened, I'd always be disappointed. But if I just go on watering and nurturing and not worrying, I suddenly notice a week or so later how much they've grown.

Allow the changes to take place via persistence and consistency. Don't panic about the everyday fluctuations we naturally have. For example, when it comes to weight, you don't weigh exactly the same all the time. Remember in chapter 2 how we established a target weight *range*—not a target weight—which is much more reasonable? These daily ups and downs are perfectly normal. Give yourself at least six weeks between retests to allow for your body to respond.

Time to Plunge

Be prepared to plunge in and go for the things for which you've been sitting on the edge. Reaching a plateau is the perfect time for recommitment. It's the time when we feel like "throwing the baby out with the bathwater," when we start to make breakthroughs. Think of it as the quiet before the storm. Don't wait for the storm to happen. That storm is going to be created by you, your commitment, and your energy. My friend David Jaynes, who was a quarterback for the Kansas City Chiefs, once said to me: "The people who get above-normal returns on their life are the people who are willing to pay the price. It's not about luck. It's about hard work and commitment."

∾

The point is, not to focus on muscle groups or obsess about specific kinds of foods to deny yourself. It's to create a new attitude about health and fitness and about yourself, your physical and spiritual selves working together harmoniously, improving together.
To become the best we can be,
a program for fitness can't be just be a fad …
—Cher

Notes

Notes

Notes

Notes

Notes

Bibliography

American Council on Exercise. *Personal Trainer Manual: The Resource for Fitness Instructors*, 1991.

Clark, Nancy, M.S., R.D. *Sports Nutrition Guide Book.* Champaign, Illinois: Leisure Press, 1990.

Editors of the Wellness Cooking School and the University of California, Berkeley. *The Wellness Low Fat Cookbook.* Rebus, Random House, 1993.

Field, Joanna. *Each Day a New Beginning.* San Francisco: Harper/Hazelden Books, 1982.

Haas, Robert, M.S. *Cher: Forever Fit.* New York: Bantam Books, 1991.

Hazelden Foundation. *Seasons of the Heart.* New York: HarperCollins Publishers, 1993.

Heyward, Vivian H., Ph.D. *Advanced Fitness Assessment and Exercise Prescription.* Champaign, Illinois: Human Kinetics Books, 1991.

Jordan, Peg, R.N., Ed. *Fitness Theory and Practice.* Sherman Oaks, California: Aerobics and Fitness Association of America and Reebok University Press, 1993.

Kashiwa, Anne, and James Rippe, M.D. *Rockport's Fitness Walking for Women.* New York: The Putnam Publishing Group, 1987.

Kravitz, Len. *Anybody's Guide to Total Fitness.* Dubuque, Iowa: Kendall/Hunt Publishing Company, 1986.

Margen, Sheldon, M.D. *The University of California at Berkeley: The Wellness Encyclopedia of Food and Nutrition.* Rebus, Random House, 1992.

McCardle, William D., Frank I. Katch, and Victor L. Katch. *Exercise Physiology: Energy, Nutrition, and Human Performance.* Philadelphia: Lea and Febiger, 1986.

Rippe, James M., M.D., and William Southmayd, M.D. *The Sports Performance Factors.* New York: The Putnam Publishing Group, 1986.

Sammann, Patricia. *YMCA Healthy Back Book.* Champaign, Illinois: Human Kinetics Publishers, 1994.

Schaef, Anne Wilson. *Meditations for Women Who Do Too Much.* San Francisco: Harper, 1990.

Simon, Harvey B., M.D., and Steven R. Levisohn, M.D. *The Athlete Within: A Personal Guide to Total Fitness.* Boston: Little, Brown and Company, 1987.

Stern, Ellen Sue. *Running On Empty: Meditations for Indispensable Women.* New York: Bantam Books, 1992.

Sweetgall, Robert, James Rippe, M.D., and Frank Katch, Ed.D., with John Dignam. *Rockport's Fitness Walking.* New York: The Putnam Publishing Group, 1985.

Sweetgall, Robert, James Rippe, M.D., and Frank Katch, Ed.D., with John Dignam. *Fitness Walking.* New York: The Putnam Publishing Group, 1985.

Wescott, Wayne. *Be Strong: Strength Training for Muscular Fitness for Men and Women.* Dubuque: Wm. C. Brown, Publishers, 1993.